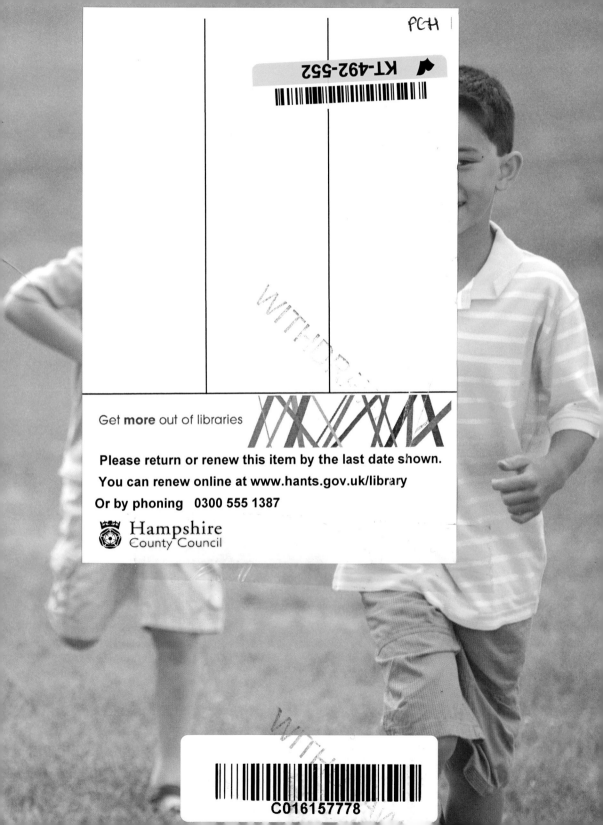

PCH

KT-492-552

FIT FOOD FOR KIDS
A DIET PLAN FOR HEALTH AND WEIGHT CONTROL

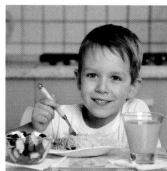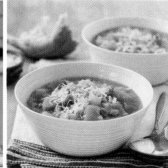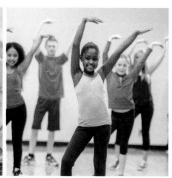

The fuss-free parental guide to getting your children moving,
motivated and eating well

Expert dietary advice for safe and sensible weight management,
with more than 100 tempting recipes

Step-by-step exercise routines and helpful menu and exercise planners

KIM DAVIES

LORENZ BOOKS

This edition is published by Lorenz Books, an imprint of Anness Publishing Ltd, 108 Great Russell Street, London WC1B 3NA; info@anness.com

www.lorenzbooks.com; www.annesspublishing.com; twitter: @Anness_Books

If you like the images in this book and would like to investigate using them for publishing, promotions or advertising, please visit our website www.practicalpictures.com for more information.

Publisher: Joanna Lorenz
Senior Editor and Designer: Lucy Doncaster
Illustrator: Georgie Fearns
Consultant Nutritionist: Penny Doyle
Production Controller: Pirong Wang

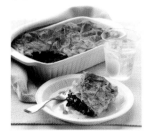

PUBLISHER'S NOTE
Although the advice and information in this book are believed to be accurate and true at the time of going to press, neither the authors nor the publisher can accept any legal responsibility or liability for any errors or omissions that may have been made nor for any inaccuracies nor for any loss, harm or injury that comes about from following instructions or advice in this book. The reader should not regard the recommendations, ideas and techniques in this book as substitutes for the advice of a medical practitioner or other qualified professional.

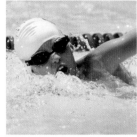

Picture credits: iStock: 4, 5, 6, 7, 8, 9, 10, 11, 12, 13, 14, 15, 16, 19, 21, 22, 23b, 24, 25, 27, 28, 29, 30, 31, 34, 36, 37, 42, 45, 46, 48, 51, 52, 54, 55, 56, 57, 58, 59, 60, 61, 62, 80, 94; Lucy Doncaster: 47.

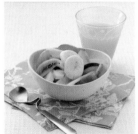

COOK'S NOTES
• Food allergies and intolerances are on the increase, especially in children under five. If your child has special dietary requirements then you should follow the guidance provided by your doctor when preparing food. If you are cooking for other children or giving a children's party, it is best to ask the parents if any of the children have special requirements and avoid using nuts altogether.
• Bracketed terms in the book are intended for American readers.
• For all recipes, quantities are given in metric and imperial measures and, where appropriate, in standard cups and spoons. Follow one set of measures, not a mixture, because they are not interchangeable.
• Standard spoon and cup measures should be level. 1 tsp = 5ml, 1 tbsp = 15ml, 1 cup = 250ml/8fl oz.
• Australian standard tablespoons are 20ml. Australian readers should use 3 tsp in place of 1 tbsp for measuring small quantities.
• American pints are 16fl oz/2 cups. American readers should use 20fl oz/ 2.5 cups in place of 1 pint when measuring liquids.
• Electric oven temperatures in this book are for conventional ovens. When using a fan oven, the temperature will probably need to be reduced by about 10–20°C/ 20–40°F. Since ovens vary, you should check the manufacturer's instruction book for guidance.
• The nutritional analysis given for each recipe, unless otherwise stated, is calculated per portion (i.e. serving or item). If the recipe gives a range, such as Serves 4–6, then the nutritional analysis will be for the smaller size, i.e. 6 servings. The analysis does not include optional ingredients, such as salt added to taste.
• Medium (US large) eggs are used unless otherwise stated in the recipe. Ideally, you should use free-range eggs whenever possible.

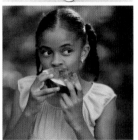

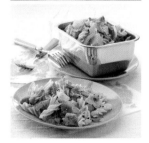

CONTENTS

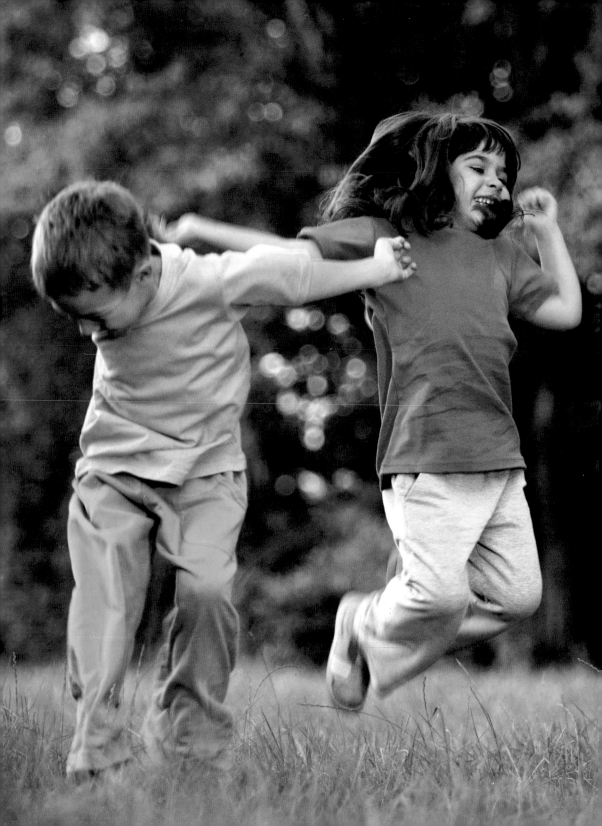

INTRODUCTION

This is a book with a very simple message: that the best way to stay well throughout your lifetime is to eat healthily and be active. We all think that we are aware of this already – but the fact is that the message is not being heard. We can be certain that this simple truth has been lost because the statistics show incontrovertibly that an ever-greater percentage of the population is overweight. Most alarmingly, the children of the current generation are more likely to be obese than in any previous one. The health implications of this for the future are enormous and worrying.

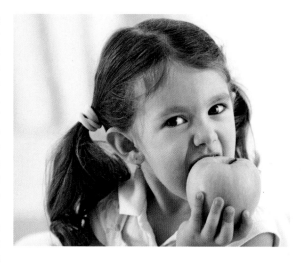

This book is not about dieting, and is not about parenting. It is about how you as a parent can shape your family's habits in such a way as to keep yourself and your children in the best possible health – because there's no doubt that children have access to a vast array of unhealthy food, and there is a huge industry dedicated to persuading them to eat it. We can't easily stop that, but we, their parents, are the biggest influence in our children's early years. This is the time to lay the foundations of healthy habits that will stand them in good stead for a lifetime.

Providing your children with nutritious food and the chance to do regular exercise not only promotes their health now, but also in the future.

Maintaining a healthy weight is key to wellness. Children who are neither overweight nor underweight tend to be fitter, have higher self-esteem and are better able to learn. They are less likely to have serious health problems, such as diabetes and heart disease, both in childhood and in later life, and there is more of a chance that they will go on to maintain a healthy weight when they are older and in charge of their own nutrition.

If your children are in good physical shape, then you can help them stay that way. And if they are underweight or overweight, then you can assist them with that too. Encouraging your child to eat a varied diet and be active will help them reach and maintain a healthy weight at any age. That's what I hope this book will achieve – helping families to live in a way that supports their well-being and ultimately their happiness.

HEALTHY KIDS, HEALTHY WEIGHT

Until recent years, maintaining a healthy weight was fairly easy for most people. Our daily lives were active and we ate a more natural diet. Most of our food was cooked from scratch, and we consumed just enough to satisfy ourselves.

But little by little, our habits have changed. Today's busy lives encourage us to take shortcuts that have impacted on our weight and health, almost without us noticing. And there is no doubt about it: people are getting bigger – obesity rates have tripled since the 1980s. In the USA, around three out of every four men (75 per cent) and three out of every five women (60 per cent) are overweight or obese. More than a third of American children are now classed as overweight or obese, and over a third of girls and a quarter of boys in the UK weigh more than is healthy.

Children are designed to run around, not to sit for hours, so set limits on your family's screentime.

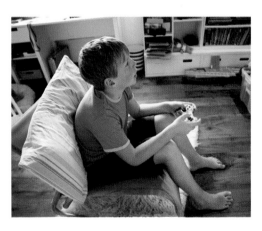

WHY ARE OUR CHILDREN GETTING BIGGER?

There's no great secret as to why this is happening – our children, like most of us, are spending many more hours sitting still in front of a screen, and less time running around. And – as every parent knows – there is junk food available wherever you turn. In the past, most families came together to eat home-cooked food every night. Nowadays, we are much more likely to eat out, or to rely on quick-to-prepare processed food. Our children (and us adults) are consuming more unhealthy food than their bodies can easily cope with, and the result is a less healthy, bigger body.

WHY DOES WEIGHT MATTER?

Being overweight makes day-to-day activities harder to manage and can make a child feel self-conscious and unhappy. It also increases the risk of:

Type 2 diabetes This form of diabetes used to be known as adult-onset diabetes, but is now increasingly affecting children and teenagers. It is thought that one in three American children born in 2000 will go on to develop diabetes caused by weight problems.

Heart disease Hardening of the arteries (atherosclerosis), which is a major cause of heart disease, may start in childhood and adolescence.

WHAT YOU CAN DO

1 Offer nutritious food, including healthy snacks and drinks, in sensible portions.

2 Provide opportunities for your child to be active. The recommended amount is 60 minutes a day.

3 Limit screentime to no more than two hours a day (nothing for the under-threes).

4 Prioritize good sleeping habits – tired children are much more likely to want high-fat, high-sugar foods.

5 Lead by example. If you have a balanced, healthy lifestyle, then your children are more likely to opt for one, too.

6 Make sharing food joyful. Beware of turning food into a battleground or source of shame.

7 Eat as a family – it's one of the most effective ways to instil good eating habits.

8 Accept and love your kids as they are. Weight is only one aspect of who a person is – help your child feel good about themselves.

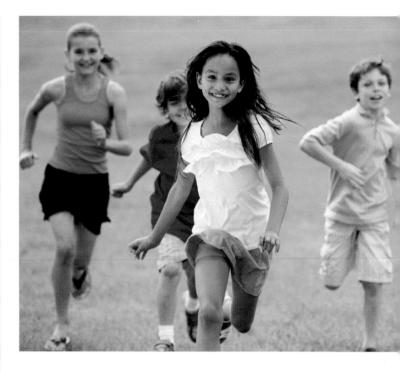

Active children are generally healthy children, and it is our role as parents to facilitate exercise and feed them a balanced diet.

High blood pressure This puts pressure on the heart, and is much more likely to affect children who are overweight.

Early puberty Overweight girls may reach puberty earlier, and are more likely to develop irregular menstruation and fibroids later in life.

Obstructive sleep apnoea This disorder, in which breathing is interrupted during sleep, may lead to heart failure. It is linked to excess weight.

Asthma Overweight children are more likely to develop asthma, a life-threatening condition that makes exercise more difficult.

Children who are overweight are more likely to develop into overweight adults. Poor diet and an inactive lifestyle become deep-rooted habits. They are also at increased risk of stroke, cancer and cardiovascular disease. It's much harder to lose weight as an adult if you have been overweight as a child, too.

WHAT IS A HEALTHY WEIGHT?

Children's bodies come in all shapes and sizes. Some will naturally be more slender or else broader than others – in just the same way that some are taller or shorter.

Teenage girls in particular will experience many changes during puberty, and some weight gain is perfectly healthy and normal as their bodies grow and develop.

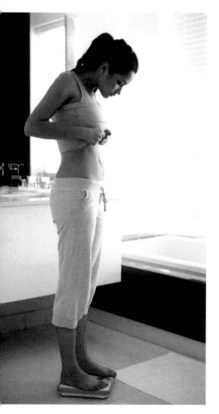

Children's bodies are constantly changing as they grow, so it is not easy to work out whether they are a healthy weight. A researcher from the University of Nebraska-Lincoln looked at 69 studies of children, and concluded that 50 per cent of parents underestimated their child's weight. And, interestingly, although US obesity rates have tripled in the last 30 years, there has been no change in the number of parents who see their children as being overweight. It seems that our perception of what a normal weight looks like has shifted as overweight people have become more prevalent in our society. This may also explain the findings of another study, which found that parents of some healthy-weight children wrongly believed them to be underweight.

THE BMI TOOL

The best way to check whether a child is a healthy weight is to use the BMI tool. This stands for Body Mass Index, and is a number that uses a person's weight and height to work out how much body fat they have. Too much body fat increases your child's risk of certain illness and other health problems, while too little can also be an issue. The BMI is a general way of checking whether a person falls within a healthy body mass range.

In adults, BMI in conjunction with waist circumference is an indicator of a person's weight, and how much over or under their ideal they are. Although it's not an exact science, a score of between 20 and 25 is considered healthy, regardless of gender, though other medical factors are considered.

A child's BMI is more complicated, because their ratio of body fat changes as they grow. For example, it is normal for a two-year-old to have a protruding belly, and weight gain is a natural part of puberty. For this reason, health professionals monitor children's height and weight from toddlerhood onwards, plotting the results on a chart that gives their BMI-for-age.

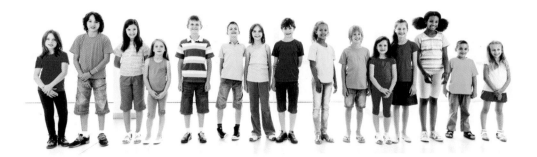

The phrase 'one size fits all' couldn't be more wrong when it comes to a child's weight. Factors such as height, gender, muscle mass and body-fat ratio all have an effect and should be taken into consideration.

CHECKING THE BMI

Ideally, you might ask a health professional to check your child's weight and BMI, but if this is not practical you can do it yourself using the guidance on the next page. Doing this regularly will help you understand whether your child is gaining weight in a natural way, or whether there has been a sudden change. Even then, you should bear in mind that children have growth spurts, when they can gain weight or increase in height rapidly, so there may be no cause for alarm.

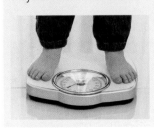

BMI-FOR-AGE

A child's BMI needs to be assessed according to their age – the BMI-for-age – and then plotted on a graph to compare it with average BMIs of other children of the same age and sex to establish the BMI percentile. A BMI-for-age percentile of 60 per cent means that 60 per cent of children of the same age, sex and height will have a BMI lower than this, and 40 per cent will have a higher one.

0–5 percentile – underweight
5–85 percentile – healthy weight
85–95 percentile – overweight
95–100 percentile – very overweight/obese

HOW RELIABLE IS THE BMI?

The BMI is a reliable indicator of the amount of fat in the body for children over the age of two years. It is not perfect, however, because muscle weighs more than fat, meaning that a very muscular child may show up as having a high BMI even though their actual proportion of body fat is comparatively low. In addition, it is more difficult to judge whether a child is overweight when their body is going through a period of rapid growth. As a result, some experts think that it is better to test children for fitness rather than BMI. That said, a child with a high BMI will usually have a high proportion of body fat, and in most cases it is the best weight-assessment tool that we have.

YOUR CHILD'S BMI

Your doctor will work out your child's BMI-for-age for you, but if you want to do it at home, you will first need to measure and weigh your child accurately. You can then use an online calculator or the BMI formula given here to work it out.

The easiest way to calculate your child's BMI-for-age at home is to use an online calculator: see the UK's NHS website, the Mayo Clinic website, or simply search for 'online BMI calculator'. All you need to do is enter an accurate height and weight for your child, together with their age and sex. The calculator will give you your child's BMI-for-age, and will tell you whether the results indicate that your child is a healthy weight, underweight, overweight or very overweight/obese. Apps such as BMI Calculator work in the same way.

The BMI provides a useful way of determining whether a child is within a healthy weight range for their age, gender and height.

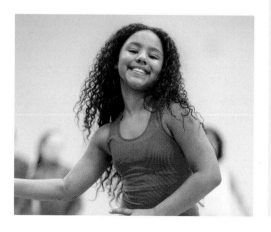

BMI FORMULAS
Alternatively, you can use one of the following formulas to calculate the BMI:

Metric
Weight in kilograms/height in metres squared

Imperial
Weight in pounds x 703/height in inches squared

To give you a rough idea of whether your child's BMI indicates that they may be overweight or very overweight/obese, compare it with these BMI figures, which are based on children of average height for their age:

Girls

age	overweight	very overweight/obese
2	18	19.1
5	16.8	18.3
8	18.3	20.7
13	23.8	28.3

Boys

age	overweight	very overweight/obese
2	18.2	19.3
5	16.8	17.9
8	18.7	21.2
13	23	27

WEIGHING YOUR CHILD

Use digital scales, and place them on a hard, level floor.

• Ask your child to remove shoes and heavy clothing, such as overcoats and sweaters.

• Have him or her stand on the scales, feet in the centre on either side of the display.

• Make a note of the weight, including the decimal fraction (eg 21.5kg or 47.5lb).

MEASURING YOUR CHILD'S HEIGHT

Your child will need to stand on a hard floor and against a flat wall.

• Ask your child to remove shoes, bulky clothing and hair accessories that prevent the head from resting against the wall.

• Get him or her to stand up straight against the wall, feet together, shoulders level and arms by the sides. The head, shoulders, buttocks and heels should be touching the wall (as far as your child's shape allows).

• Ask your child to look straight ahead, eyes parallel to the floor.

• Place a flat object (such as a hard-backed book) at right angles to the wall and slide it down to rest on the top of your child's head. Check he or she is looking straight ahead.

• Using a pencil, mark where the bottom edge of the object meets the wall.

• Measure from the floor to the mark, using a metal tape measure.

• Make a note of the measurement to the nearest 1mm or ⅛in.

DOES MY CHILD NEED TO LOSE ANY WEIGHT?

In most cases of overweight children, the goal is not to lose weight but to maintain their current weight. This means that they will slim down gradually as they get older, and grow taller.

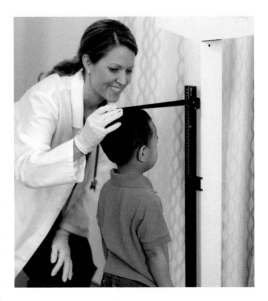

Your child's height and weight may be monitored by your doctor or a health worker at school.

Children who are underweight generally catch up when they finish puberty – it is rare for them to be advised to put on weight.

If a child is seriously overweight – and especially if he or she has weight-related health issues – then a doctor may recommend weight loss, but this should be very gradual and only attempted with professional health advice.

Sometimes an issue with weight is linked to an underlying health problem or perhaps an eating disorder that needs treatment. For example, gaining excess weight may be the result of a hormonal imbalance or an underactive thyroid, or it may be linked to medication that a child is taking. You should see a doctor to rule this out.

However, most often excess weight is caused by eating too much of the wrong foods and not being sufficiently active.

IT'S A FAMILY AFFAIR

There's compelling evidence to suggest that the best way to help a child maintain a healthy weight is to involve the whole family. A 'do as I do' not a 'do as I say' approach works best.

Our children don't live in isolation, they live in a family, and so it is important that the choices we make apply to each member of that family. It's much easier to encourage a child who is overweight to be more active or to eat healthy snacks instead of crisps or potato chips, say, if everyone else in the family is treated the same way. This might sound unfair, but if one person in a family has a weight problem, it is unlikely that other members are eating healthily. And ultimately, having a healthy lifestyle will benefit everyone even if they miss the junk food.

WHAT PARENTS DO

As parents, we all wonder how much influence we have on our children. They can seem such strong individuals, and there are so many other factors that work on them away from the home. But the fact is that parents are in the best possible position to nudge children towards a healthier lifestyle. Because as parents:

We are providers of food Children don't make their own decisions about what they eat. Most households have a 'nutritional gatekeeper' who plans, buys and provides the food. This person influences the meals served at home and makes choices about any number of smaller things, such as whether the family eats round a table or in front of the TV; and he or she selects foods for packed lunches and picnics. One study found that 72 per cent of what children eat is influenced by the home's gatekeeper.

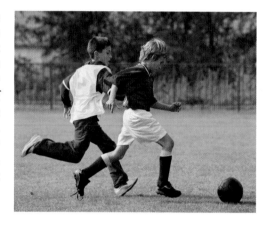

Parents have to be prepared to spend time and money in order that children can participate in team sports.

We are activity facilitators If our children want to go to football practice and Sunday matches, if they want to start gymnastics or baseball, then parents are usually going to have to pay for the classes and the kit, and get them wherever they want to go. Likewise, we decide when they are old enough to walk to school alone, and take them out for a run-around or to the swimming pool. And we control the amount of screentime our children have.

We are role models Children instinctively look to their parents to show them how to make sense of the world, particularly when they are young. In one study, researchers looking at more than 550 families found that the quantity of fruit and vegetables eaten by parents was the strongest indicator of the amount eaten by their offspring. The message is clear: if you want your child to live healthily, you have to do so too.

We are taste-setters Research shows that a child's food preferences are shaped in the early years. Babies naturally prefer sweet and salty foods, and avoid bitter and sour flavours. The way they learn to like the latter is by being repeatedly exposed to them. By continuing to present our children with nourishing foods, we guide them towards a liking for them.

We are authorities As the adults, it is up to us to set the rules. Children are naturally primed to push against boundaries – to ask for more confectionery, or to eat in front of the TV – but the more consistent you are, the more accepting your children become. That doesn't mean being overly authoritarian – in fact, trying to force a child to act healthily often makes them more resistant. And although consistency is key, you don't need to be totally rigid: it is fine to relax the rules from time to time, and allow your children to enjoy party food or an ice cream at the park.

We are advocates We can help change the way our children are treated outside the home, too. We can lobby for changes in school meal provision, talk to the school about banning confectionery from the playground, find ways to improve outdoor spaces so our children have somewhere to play, and generally make clear what we do and don't want our children to eat.

WORKING WITH OTHER PEOPLE

Parents are not the only important people in our children's lives: grandparents, uncles and aunts, siblings, godparents, childminders, nursery workers and teachers all have a role. We may not be able to influence the way that our children's friends operate, but we can ask adult relatives and childcare providers to help support healthy habits by not giving children unhealthy treats; encourage them instead to give fruit, such as strawberries or blueberries, or non-food rewards such as stickers or magazines as a treat.

In most families there is a 'nutritional gatekeeper' who makes and implements most of the dietary decisions in a household.

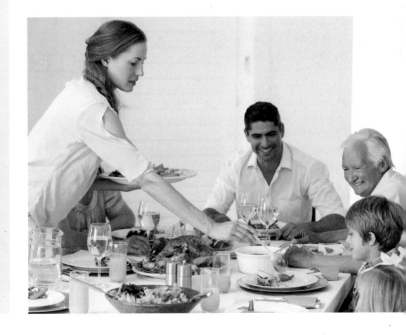

WHY DIET MATTERS

The food you eat – and how much of it you eat – has a huge impact on your well-being. A nutritious, well-balanced diet helps you to stay well, and maintain the right weight.

A healthy diet is vital – and not just to weight and health. It is linked to better performance at school and in sports, helps to balance moods, and increases energy for everyday activities.

In children, as with adults, a healthy body weight is the result of a balance between the number of calories consumed, and the number of calories burned up through activity. Calories – abbreviated to kcal – are simply a measure of the amount of energy contained in food and drink. These simple facts apply in the vast majority of cases, unless there is an underlying health problem causing a weight issue:
• A child who consumes a greater number of calories than the body uses up (burns) will put on weight. The body converts the extra calories into fat, and stores it.
• A child who consumes fewer calories than the body uses will lose weight. The body will burn up its fat stores to get the energy it needs.
• A child who consumes the same amount of calories that they need for growth and activity will maintain a stable weight.

HOW MANY CALORIES A DAY?
There are guidelines for the number of calories that men and women need per day. It's difficult to give a precise healthy daily amount of calories for children, however, because they are still growing, and they need different amounts of calories to fuel their growth at different ages and stages of development.

There really is no such thing as a perfect daily amount of calories for, say, a 10-year-old – it depends on their size, how active they are and how fast they are growing. The closest we can get is a calorie range. This is for children of average size and weight; the lower end of the range is for children who are not very active, the highest for the most active ones:

Girls
age	daily kcal requirements
2–3	1,000–1,400
4–8	1,200–1,800
9–13	1,400–2,200
14–18	1,800–2,400

By swapping fatty, sugary snacks for healthy ones, you will considerably boost your child's nutrition.

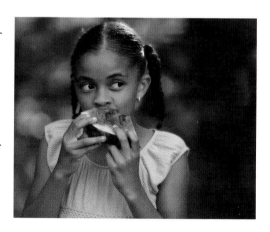

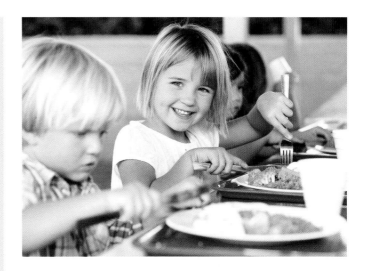

It is worth finding out what your child is eating for lunch on a daily basis at school or nursery so you can assess their daily calorie intake.

Boys

age	daily kcal requirements
2–3	1,000–1,400
4–8	1,200–2,000
9–13	1,600–2,600
14–18	2,000–3,200

These ranges can only ever be guidelines, but it can be helpful to bear them in mind when looking at what you feed your children – if they are having a high-calorie lunch, then a lower-calorie dinner might be a good idea. Calorie counts are given for the recipes in this book to help you, along with menu planners that show how you could potentially combine dishes during a day to provide a balanced diet along with a sensible number of calories.

If your child is overweight, then your instinct may be to restrict calories by giving them less to eat. But all the experts say that this is counterproductive if it leaves the child hungry.

They may simply find other ways – sneakier, and less healthy still – to get the food they want. Or you may find that meals and snacks turn into a battleground, which sets up unhealthy attitudes towards food. A more sensible course of action – one agreed on by most experts in child weight control – is to switch the diet to a more healthy one that includes fewer unhealthy fats and sugars and more nutritious, sustaining alternatives.

A gentle approach means that your child should maintain rather than lose weight. This is better for him or her (unless your child is specifically advised to lose weight under the guidance of a doctor), and you should find that the child slims down naturally as he or she grows. Simultaneously increasing the amount of exercise they take will also naturally burn more calories, which will aid the levelling-off of their weight, as well as burning excess fat and improving fitness.

MAKING HEALTHY CHOICES

All the experts agree that having a good balanced diet is key to maintaining a healthy weight. And it is not just what and how much you eat that matters – when and how you eat are important too.

There is so much advice about healthy eating that parents are often confused about what to feed their children. In general terms, however, it is best to eat fresh, home-made food using good-quality ingredients and to reserve very high-fat or calorific foods for special occasions. The principles outlined in the box opposite can be applied to most diets, and pages 18–21 look in detail at the different food groups and children's dietary requirements.

START EARLY, EAT BREAKFAST

Having regular meals is an important part of healthy eating and breakfast really is the most important meal of the day, especially for young ones. Children who have breakfast have been shown to do better in class and the playground – a good breakfast improves concentration and problem-solving abilities, as well as boosting hand-to-eye coordination.

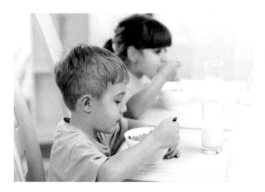

Eating a healthy breakfast helps with weight control, too, since studies show that people who eat breakfast usually make healthier food choices throughout the day and are less likely to snack. Your metabolism slows down at night when you are at rest. Having breakfast – breaking your fast – in the morning gets it going again so that your body can start burning calories efficiently.

Good breakfasts should include some wholegrain carbohydrate such as oats, or wholemeal or whole-wheat bread or cereal, which are nutrient-dense and provide slow-release glucose for the brain and muscles. Small portions of protein such as eggs, lean meat, fish or baked beans are also good for the hungrier child as they create a feeling of fullness.

SNACKTIME

Offering healthy snacks, such as fruits and vegetables and wholegrains (oatcakes and rice cakes), is a good way of increasing the amount of nutrients your children get. And because these foods are filling, they reduce cravings for junk foods: snacks that provide only 'empty calories', so called because they contain energy without many nutrients. If you do give your child crisps or potato chips, don't allow them to have an adult portion – put half in a bowl and save the rest. Plain popcorn is a better choice.

Breakfast is a very important meal, especially for children, and will set them up for the day.

HEALTHY EATING PRINCIPLES

These guidelines cover the main foods that should be consumed on a weekly basis, and those that should be minimized. Young children and those with special diets and medical conditions should adhere to specific medical advice.

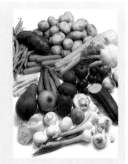

Have more

Fruits and vegetables Have at least five a day, ideally seven or more. Try to 'eat a rainbow', offering a wide range of differently coloured fruit and vegetables, and at least two types of vegetable at dinner.

Wholegrains Starchy foods (such as grains and potatoes) should form the basis of your meals. Go for wholemeal or whole-wheat bread and rice and whole oats, since these contain nutrient-rich germ and fibre-rich bran, which are removed from refined grains (white bread and rice). A diet high in wholegrains is better for adults and children over five (younger children can't process too much fibre) because it aids digestion and – crucially – helps you feel full up.

Fish and other lean high-protein foods Aim for two servings of fish a week (one of which should be oily fish), and choose lean meats and poultry, eggs, nuts, lentils and beans rather than hamburgers, sausages and bacon.

Milk and water These are the best drinks for children. Give those older than two years semi-skimmed milk; under-twos need full-fat (whole) milk.

Have less

Sugar Cut back on the cakes, confectionery and cookies that your children have. They provide many empty calories for very little nutritional gain, and sugar is also responsible for the increase in dental disease that is being seen in children. Go for more natural treats, such as home-made cakes or fruit ice cream or sorbet, and good-quality chocolate. These at least contain some nutritional benefit and are likely to be lower in sugar. Experiment by cutting the sugar in baking recipes – in some you can reduce the sugar by up to a third without adversely affecting their taste or texture.

Fizzy drinks Sugary drinks are a major cause of obesity in children and are a totally unnecessary food choice. Make them an occasional indulgence, at most. Water is best.

Processed meats Burgers, sausages, bacon, salami and pies are high in fat and salt, and the method by which they are processed may be linked to heart disease.

High-fat foods Butter, cream, full-fat cheese, cakes, crisps or potato chips, French fries, deep-fried foods and chocolate should all be eaten in moderation.

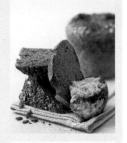

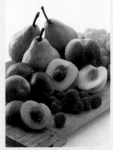

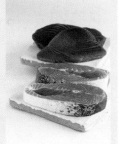

A BALANCED DIET

Being aware that you should have a balanced diet is one thing; knowing how to eat is a different matter. But eating well is a skill that you can learn – and involves just a few simple principles.

A balanced diet is one that is based on the five food groups, eaten in the right proportions. We should all have a diet that is high in fibre and low in fat. And most of what we eat should consist of cereals or other starchy foods and vegetables and fruit, with the rest consisting of dairy products and high-quality protein foods.

The food pyramid shown below is a handy visual guide to the variety and ratios of the food you should eat each day. You don't have to keep to it for every meal, of course, so long as you stick roughly to the proportions over the course of the day. Go for low-salt foods wherever possible (see box, overleaf).

THE FIVE FOOD GROUPS

Cereals and potatoes Starchy carbohydrates should be included in each meal, making up about one-third of the daily diet, and might include bread, cereals, potatoes, pasta or rice. Carbohydrates provide vital energy for busy brains and active bodies, and are not particularly high in calories so long as they are not deep-fried, or served with cheese or butter. Choose wholegrain and lower-GI options where possible. These include basmati rice, noodles, oats, sweet or new potatoes, or al dente pasta. Processed potato products, jasmine rice and white bread are all higher GI and less sustaining.

The food pyramid is a useful visual representation of how the ratios of the food groups should appear over the course of a day.

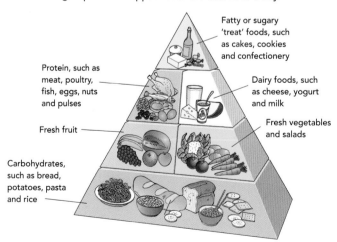

Fatty or sugary 'treat' foods, such as cakes, cookies and confectionery

Protein, such as meat, poultry, fish, eggs, nuts and pulses

Dairy foods, such as cheese, yogurt and milk

Fresh fruit

Fresh vegetables and salads

Carbohydrates, such as bread, potatoes, pasta and rice

LOW-GI FOODS

Wholegrains have a low glycaemic index (GI). This indicates the speed with which the glucose a food contains is released into your bloodstream. The GI runs from 0 to 100; the lower the number the better, because it means that the glucose is released gradually, staving off hunger. For example, cornflakes have a high GI of 93 while porridge is 40. Low-GI foods are generally high in fibre, too.

FOOD AND THE UNDER-TWOS

Children under the age of two have small stomachs so need smaller and more frequent meals. They also need more fat, which is essential for brain growth, so it is important that young children have full-fat dairy foods, including plenty of whole milk, and healthy-fat foods, such as meat, oily fish, avocados and the dark meat of poultry. Sugary or processed foods should be kept to the minimum or, ideally, not given at all. After their second birthday, a child can move towards the same diet as the rest of the family.

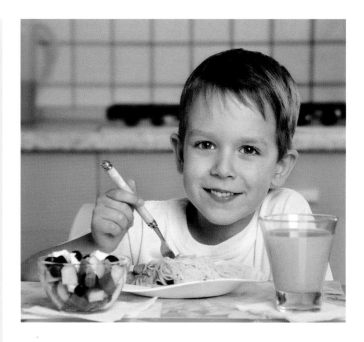

The majority of our diet should be made up of fresh fruit and vegetables, carbohydrates, protein and a little healthy fat.

Vegetables and fruits Give your children at least five (ideally seven) portions of vegetables and fruit a day (especially dark green, red and orange veg). Fresh, frozen, canned and dried forms all count, but dried fruit should only be given once a day because it is high in sugar.

Lower-fat dairy products Children require three servings of calcium per day (one more than adults), to build strong bones. A serving is 200ml/7fl oz/scant 1 cup of milk, a chunk of cheese (enough to fill a sandwich) or a small pot of yogurt. Low-fat milk and yogurt actually contain more calcium than high-fat versions.

High-protein foods Protein is essential for muscle-growth and is an important source of key nutrients. Choose lean cuts of meat, poultry, fish, pulses, nuts or eggs, and offer two servings of fish (one oily) a week. Most children get sufficient protein, but vegetarians need to take care that they receive enough. Be aware that vegetarian sources of protein don't contain all the nutrients (amino acids) that we need; if you don't eat much meat or fish, make sure that each meal combines at least two of the following foods: dairy products, grains, and beans or lentils.

Fats and sugars We all need essential fats in our diets, but try to eat more from oils, spreads, nuts and fish rather than animal fats such as fatty meats, hard cheese and butter. Sugar is a natural part of foods such as dairy, fruits and vegetables, but foods that have added sugar should be limited. Check the label: a food that has more than 22.5g/1oz sugar per 100g/3½oz serving is far too sweet.

HOW TO ENCOURAGE GOOD EATING HABITS

Children aren't always amenable to eating healthily, but there are subtle ways in which you can encourage them.

Most children do eat some vegetables – 90 per cent eat them every day, according to one US survey – but they generally don't eat enough and teenagers tend to eat less than younger children. Here are some ways to up the vegetable and fruit content of their diets:

• A lot of children are interested in cooking, and they may be more excited about healthy food if they have had a hand in helping to prepare it. Growing cress or tomatoes is a simple way they can learn more about where vegetables come from, or you might like to do 'pick your own' or visit a farm. Older children and teens may be able to cook a family meal.

• Research shows that a child may need to be offered a particular food 10 times or more before they start to like it. Praise them for trying – and offer them a sticker as a reward. Only present one new food at a time, alongside tried-and-tested favourites. Serve vegetables with every meal and let them see you enjoying them.

• Add finely chopped courgette or zucchini in bolognese, or grated carrot or shredded spinach in a tomato sauce for pasta.

• Mash sweet potatoes or swede (rutabaga) instead of or in combination with white potatoes. This can be used in the same way as mashed potato, but contains more vitamins.

• Serve lightly cooked or raw vegetables, such as sugarsnap peas, baby carrots or sweet (bell) pepper with a dip such as hummus or plain yogurt (not mayonnaise).

• Team vegetables with a food your child likes – peanut butter spread on celery, low-fat cheese sprinkled over broccoli.

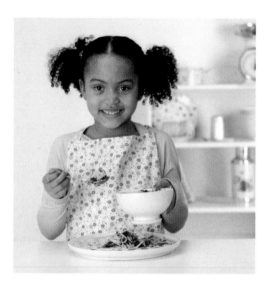

Children are more likely to eat vegetables if they have helped to prepare and cook them.

• Go for peer pressure. Invite one of your child's friends, who you know is more adventurous, over for dinner. Serve a vegetable without comment and see whether your child tries it.

• Make up a box of cut vegetables and fruit, and leave it in the refrigerator so it is to hand for snacks. Or put out a plate of chopped vegetables and salad when you are preparing dinner. A pot of frozen peas or corn can really appeal, too.

• Serve some meals buffet-style, and include vegetable options: a bowl of green beans, another of cherry tomatoes, baby corn, etc. Children often prefer their food to be separate, so they can pick and choose what they want.

PLAY WITH YOUR FOOD!

Making food fun means it is less intimidating for smaller children, and more appealing to experiment with. Try these ideas to get them enjoying their veg:

BE SALT-AWARE

Many people eat far more salt than is good for them. However, liking salty foods is a learned preference – if you don't have it, you won't miss it. High salt intake is associated with high blood pressure and it has been linked to obesity, because it encourages children to increase their consumption of sweet drinks. Children's bodies are not good at processing salt, so don't add it to their food.

The guideline maximum amounts for children are:
1–3 years 2g/day
4–6 years 3g/day
7–10 years 5g/day
11 years and over 6g/day

Salt is a compound called sodium chloride, but food labels give only the amount of sodium, not the chloride component, per 100g serving. If you want to work out the salt content, multiply the sodium by 2.5. If you are using stock or bouillon cubes, sauces, or processed foods, opt for the low-salt versions and do not add any extra salt. Flavoured oils, garlic, herbs, spices and lemon juice are all handy salt-free flavourings.

• Arrange vegetables into a face – for some reason, small children find this hilarious.
• Call broccoli 'trees' – hold up a small floret and say, 'Here's a tree in summer,' then bite off the top and say, 'Here's a tree in winter,' before chomping the stalk ('and here is the woodsman to chop up the trunk').
• Tell your kids that their eyes flash green every time they eat a pea – ham it up so they (sort of) know you are joking.
• Challenge your child to a green-bean eating race – and let them win every time.

THE IMPORTANCE OF IRON

It's important that children get enough iron, which is needed for healthy blood, growth and development. So make sure you serve iron-rich foods, such as red meat, the dark meat of poultry, tuna and salmon. Iron is found in nuts, eggs, tofu, dried fruits, baked beans, dried beans and peas, lentils, leafy green vegetables, and fortified breakfast cereals. Serving these foods alongside ones that are rich in vitamin C (oranges, broccoli, strawberries and tomatoes) helps the body to absorb iron.

Presenting food to your children in a fun and attractive way will mean that they are more likely to want to eat it, and try new ingredients.

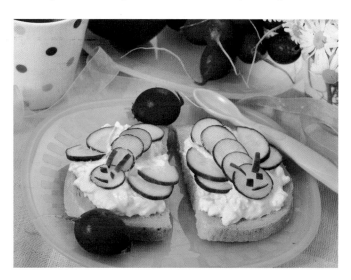

EATING OUT

We are eating more restaurant and takeaway food than ever before, and that means less control over what we consume. Here are some ways to make wise choices when you look at a menu.

We all enjoy eating out from time to time, but if you eat out a lot, you need to take into account that restaurant and takeaway foods tend to contain more sugar, salt and fat than home-cooked food. And portions are much, much bigger than they used to be. The National Heart, Blood and Lung Institute compared typical servings 20 years ago with those of today. They found that the number of calories in a typical serving of spaghetti, meatballs and tomato sauce had doubled.

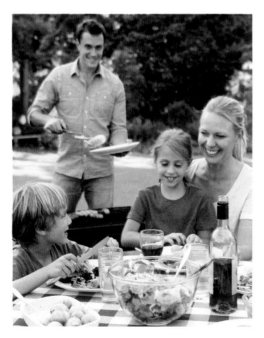

You can reduce what you eat by forgoing extras — such as bread and butter or sauces (mayonnaise or barbecue sauce can add tens of calories to your meal). If you want an appetizer, then go for soup — a study at Pennsylvania State University found that it can reduce the amount of calories eaten overall in a meal by 25 per cent. Talk to your waiter about how dishes are cooked so that you can avoid fried foods, or ask for your dish to be cooked differently. And it's always best to wait until after you have eaten your main before ordering dessert — you may not want it. Remind children (and yourself) that you don't have to finish everything. Eat slowly, and stop when you feel full.

Be particularly wary of children's menus, which often focus on high-fat foods, such as sausages, chicken nuggets and burgers. A survey of 21 outlets by the British Soil Association found that more than a third included no vegetables or salad with children's meals. Ordering a side dish of vegetables, or even bringing your own cut-up vegetables, helps to boost the meal's nutrient content. Alternatively, seek out restaurants that will do your children a smaller version of an adult meal — traditional Italian restaurants are a good bet for this; you can also ask for an extra plate and share your own meal.

Whether you're at a barbecue at a friend's house or at a restaurant or cafe, it is important to maintain the healthy diet you are implementing at home.

Steer your children (and yourself) away from the high-fat options. Here are
some healthier choices for restaurant and takeaway eating.

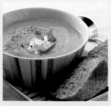
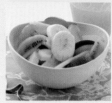

Go for	*Rather than*
vegetable soup	appetizers with cheese, pastry, meats
grilled (broiled) lean meats or fish	bacon, sausages, pies
tomato or vegetable sauces	cream or cheese sauces
steamed or boiled rice	fried rice or noodles
baked or boiled potatoes	fried potatoes, buttery mash
plain salad	salad with oil dressing, mayonnaise
fruit salad, low-fat yogurt, sorbet	ice cream, chocolate desserts, cakes
water or semi-skimmed milk	soda, squash or fruit juice

PACKED LUNCHES

Lunch accounts for between a third and half of
all calories consumed during the day, so it is
essential that it is full of nutrients. Some studies
show that school lunches are better for children
than the average packed lunch, because of the
amount of packaged foods that many parents
include in the latter. That said, packing a healthy
lunch for your child is easy, and it is a great way
to reinforce healthy-eating habits you practise at
home. Here are some tips for a healthy lunchbox:
• Use whole-wheat bread – wraps, bagels, pittas,
as well as cut bread. Watch the size – a bagel, for
example, is double the size it was 20 years ago, so
half a bagel will be enough for many children.
Use a healthy filling that provides some protein:
lean chicken, cottage cheese, tuna and corn.
• Give your child oatcakes or rice cakes instead
of a sandwich, perhaps with a little tub of lean,
low-salt, good-quality ham or chicken, a naturally
low-fat cheese (such as Edam, Emmental or
cottage cheese) – or else a dip such as hummus.

**Packing a healthy lunch for your child gives you
some control over what they eat at school.**

• Buy a wide-necked vacuum flask, and use it for
hot pasta with a tomato or pesto sauce (no added
cheese), vegetable soup or reheated leftovers.
• Include cut-up or small vegetables – carrot,
cucumber, celery, (bell) pepper, baby corn, cherry
tomatoes all work well.
• Include fresh fruit, such as cut-up pineapple,
a satsuma, grapes or cherries, and a small serving
of dried fruit, such as mango, apricots or raisins.
With a low-fat yogurt, this makes a great dessert.
• Give them a small bottle of water rather than
a sweet drink. If your children are used to having
juice, try diluting it.

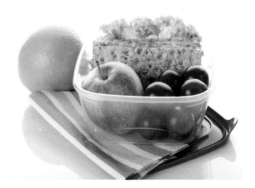

HEALTHY SHOPPING

Cooking wholesome meals is impossible if you don't have the right ingredients to hand. Healthy eating starts with making the right choices at the stores.

Supermarkets are designed to make you spend, and many of the enticing offers are for food that will do you no good at all. You have to shop, but resist the temptation to impulse-buy: when you want to eat well, the supermarket is generally not on your side.

Ideally, you should make a list and stick to it. Check your cupboards and freezer to see what you already have, work out what you are going to eat each day of the week ahead – use the menu planners on pages 38–41 – then create your shopping list. Organize it in sections: produce, meat, dairy, packaged goods, household

items etc, to help you get round the supermarket quicker – the less time you spend there the better as far as resisting temptation goes. It's a good idea to keep an ongoing list in your kitchen so that you can make a note of staple foods, such as rice and pasta, when you notice you are running low, or use an app.

WHERE TO SHOP

If at all possible, it is a good idea to do your main shop for staples online – if you don't go to the supermarket, then you can't fall prey to marketing tricks. It still helps to have made a list

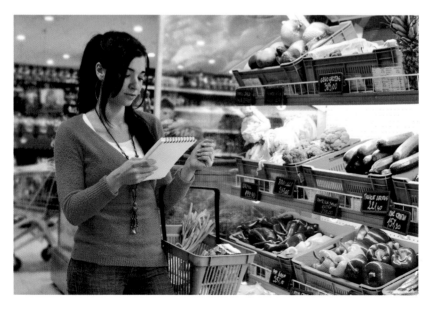

If you do need to go into a supermarket, try to go on your own, without children to distract you and cause you to impulse-buy treats to keep them happy. Write a list of all the items you need before you set out, organizing it by section, and stick to it. If you have had something to eat before you go then all the better, as you won't be tempted to buy a snack while you are in the store.

though, since internet stores also have a range of psychological ploys to get you to buy more. For fresh food, why not try a fruit-and-vegetable box, delivered to your door straight from the farm, or seek out local farmers' markets and individual stores. These often sell more local foods, and since these have travelled a shorter distance than many supermarket items, they may contain more nutrients. A farmers' market will be stocked with the kinds of nutritious foods that a healthy diet is based upon. Although each item might be more expensive than it would be in a supermarket, you may find that you don't spend more because you purchase only what you need. Buying from individual sellers is also a great way of exploring new foods – your kids may love trying stallholders' samples, too.

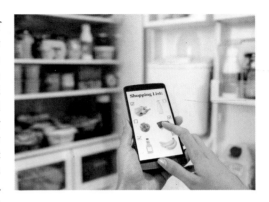

There are now numerous apps that can help you monitor your supplies and shop online in a very targeted and efficient manner.

BEAT THE SUPERMARKET

If you get your groceries from the supermarket, be sure to eat before you set out, as hunger tends to lead to impulse-buys. Shop on your own if possible – you are more likely to make impulse-purchases if you are with someone else, especially your child. If you do need to shop with your children, do it when they are not hungry or too tired, tell them beforehand that you won't be buying sugary foods, and to keep them occupied get them to pick out their preferred fruit or find items on the shelves for you.

When you are in the store, stick to the perimeter, which is usually where the healthy options are (fresh produce, meat, dairy). Make forays into the central aisles – where most packaged foods are – only to get the things you need; do not meander down the confectionery aisle.

Be label-savvy: read the packaging to check the sugar and salt content. Most ready-prepared foods have sugar in them, even seemingly healthy items such as salads and baked beans. Canned foods may contain sugar or salt. For example, tuna may be preserved in brine, oil or (the much healthier) spring water, while fruit can come in sugary syrup or natural juice.

Use a cart rather than a basket: although it might seem a good idea to have a smaller receptacle for your groceries, a study published in the *Journal of Marketing Research* found that basket-shoppers were more likely to pick up products on display when they reached the cashier; the effort of carrying a heavy basket made them reward themselves with a treat.

EAT SEASONAL, EAT LOCAL

Variety is the spice of life, so go with the seasons and try to use local ingredients where possible in order to maximize the range of nutrients your family consumes. Don't be afraid to use frozen vegetables and fruits when the fresh types are out of season; frozen ones are likely to have a higher vitamin content than their fresh counterparts if those have been flown halfway around the world.

HEALTHY COOKING

Smart cooking means preserving as many of the nutrients contained in fresh food as possible, without adding unnecessary extras such as lots of oil or butter.

Many fruits and vegetables are healthiest before they are cooked, so make raw foods a part of your diet. Salads and cut-up vegetables are an easy way to increase your fruit-and-vegetable intake. But not all foods are healthiest when raw – obviously meat, poultry and fish need cooking thoroughly, but some vegetables, including carrots, spinach, peppers and tomatoes, are also better for you when they are cooked.

In general, these are the most health-friendly ways to cook:

Steaming or boiling Steaming food in an electric steamer or on a rack or basket placed above a pan of boiling water preserves more nutrients and maintains better food colour than when the food is boiled. It's a good way to cook many vegetables, although evidence shows that carrots, courgettes (zucchini) and broccoli are more nutritious when boiled. You can steam veg or fish in a metal basket or in Chinese bamboo containers that sit on top of the pan; fish can be wrapped in foil first – add a little lemon, grated ginger, or soft-leaved herbs for flavouring.

Poaching This method involves cooking food in simmering water, milk or well-flavoured stock. It is good for fish, eggs and tender cuts of meat.

Microwaving Cooking food fast with a little water (essentially steaming it) is an effective way to maintain the nutrients. Use a lidded dish or cover with a plate rather than using clear film (plastic wrap); never put metal or foil in a microwave, or plastic that is not designed for the purpose.

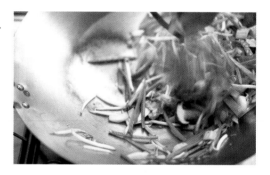

Stir-frying is one of the fastest and best ways to cook vegetables, preserving most of their nutrients.

Parcels Seafood or vegetables can be wrapped in foil or greaseproof (waxed) paper and baked in the oven. Add a little lemon and a drizzle of olive or rapeseed oil to keep it moist.

Grilling (broiling) This is a great way to maintain the juiciness of meat and vegetables, which need to be brushed with a little oil or marinated in oil, lemon and herbs/spices. Place the food on a rack so any fat drips below. Don't overcook meat – there's evidence to link regular consumption of charred meats with some cancers.

Stir-frying This method adds oil, but you only need just enough to coat the pan because the food should be cut into thin, uniform-size pieces that cook fast at high temperatures (constantly moving the food around prevents it from burning). You'll need a wok or heavy frying pan, and use vegetable or coconut oil.

Baking Many foods can be baked in the oven, including otherwise unhealthy favourites such as pizza, French fries and potato wedges. These can all easily be made and cooked at home, with minimal fat and no salt, preservatives or other undesirable additives. You can even create vegetable 'crisps' or 'chips' by thinly slicing root vegetables or beetroot (beets) and baking them at a low temperature until crispy.

However you cook your food, be sure not to overcook fruits and vegetables or you will destroy their essential nutrient content. Meat, fish and eggs need to be cooked through, and grains should be cooked so that they are tender.

THE HEALTHIEST EXTRAS

Really fresh food rarely requires any additions to make it taste good, but when you do need to add other ingredients – to cook it or to spice it up – make sure these are fresh and healthy too:

• Choose healthy fats, such as olive, coconut and other vegetable oils, rather than lard or white cooking fat, and butter.

• Use all oil in moderation – a spray bottle can help you get a very thin layer on a pan, or use kitchen paper to wipe the oil on to the pan.

• Use fresh herbs, pepper, spices and citrus fruits to add flavour to your food, rather than salt.

PORTION DISTORTION

We know that portions in restaurants and supermarkets are much, much bigger than they used to be, and there is evidence that we are serving bigger portions at home, too. Sensible portions are key to maintaining a healthy weight. But it is difficult for parents to know how much children should eat, because it varies depending on their age, size and sex. Here's another rule of thumb: get your child to make a fist and compare it with yours – it's a good indication of the proportion of an adult serving they should be eating: if their fist is two-thirds the size of yours, aim to give them two-thirds of an adult portion. Remember to offer children small portions at first and to let them ask for more if they want it.

DOUBLE UP
When cooking your family's favourite meals, double up on the quantities so that you can freeze half for a later date, if the dish will allow it. This is an easy way to ensure that you have wholesome meals on hand when you don't have time to cook.

By making pizzas at home you can pile on healthy toppings and omit or minimize high-fat and high-salt alternatives.

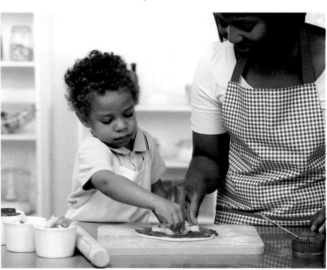

THE PSYCHOLOGY OF FOOD

Our attitude towards food plays a huge part in how we eat. Understanding the psychological significance of food can help you and your children adopt a balanced approach.

Food is more than energy: it plays a major role in human life. It is through food that we first bond with our mother; food gives us our first experience of sharing with others; and food is central to socializing and celebrating – it brings us together.

Many parents worry about their children's eating habits – poor table manners, playing with food, and suchlike. It is important to realize that food is one of the few things over which a child can exert control. They may reject some just to try out their independence muscles, for example. Young children naturally become more selective in their choice of food after the age of one – physiologically, this is the age when they become mobile; it is important that they have the ability to spit out or reject things that they come across. By the age of two, most children like to have a diet of safe, familiar favourites, so it is common for them to start rejecting foods that they previously liked.

These behaviours often disappear as the child grows older, and generally they don't have a negative impact on growth and development. They are only an issue if they are causing the child or parent anxiety, or if the child isn't eating a sufficiency of the right kinds of foods to keep healthy. However, parents often find themselves coaxing a child to eat more, threatening or force-feeding, or bribing with treats. But lavishing extra attention on a child who doesn't eat can tempt them to continue with the behaviour all the more, while tension at mealtimes may cause anxiety. A parent's excessive concern may be a factor in a child developing an eating disorder, or – more commonly – it can help create unhealthy attitudes towards food.

EMOTIONAL EATING

In an ideal world we would eat enough to nourish our body, but not to overwhelm it. Our food would be tasty and wholesome, so that it was both enjoyable to eat and good for us.

Children love to serve themselves, so offer a range of healthy foods and let them decide what to eat.

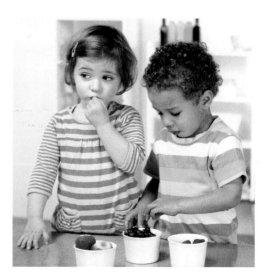

WHEN TO SEE
A DOCTOR
Eating issues with children are
often a phase, but see your
doctor if your child:

• Loses weight (it is very rare
for a healthy child to lose
weight, since they are growing
all the time).
• Starts gaining weight at a
much faster rate than they
have done in the past.
• Frequently makes negative
comments about their weight
or their appearance.

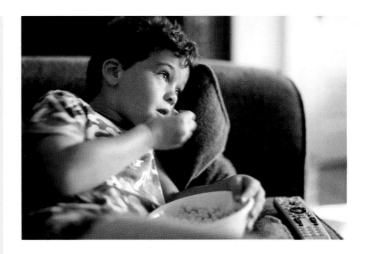

Humans often snack when they are bored, so try to occupy your
children and impose a 'no snacks on the sofa' policy, for all the family.

But modern life disrupts our natural patterns of eating. We may eat on the run, skip breakfast in the morning, swallow our food without properly chewing it, or keep ourselves going with high-fat, high-sugar snacks. And we eat when we are not hungry: for comfort if we feel sad or lonely, or for distraction when we are a bit bored. Or we don't eat because we are stressed or upset, or trying to lose weight. We may talk negatively about our bodies and our food intake.

These are the distorted attitudes towards food that many adults display. Children take their lead from their families, so such behaviours may shape their attitudes. And children are also taking in information from television programmes, from other adults and from their peers. Children are more susceptible to advertising than adults, because they find it harder to distinguish fact from fiction: they may really believe that a fizzy drink will make them more popular.

The prospect of instilling a healthier attitude towards food in your children can feel quite daunting. But remember, you have more influence than you might think, and some straightforward measures can help you to build the foundation of healthy eating habits:
• Don't comment negatively on your body or those of other people. In particular, don't criticize your child's body or weight.
• Don't talk about food in terms of it being fattening or 'naughty'.
• Eat together – food should be enjoyed communally whenever possible.
• Let children serve themselves, but encourage them to take small portions at first. Many small children will eat only as much as they need.
• Don't have a clean-your-plate rule. This overrides a child's sense of fullness, which helps regulate food intake.
• Never force-feed, threaten or bribe a child to eat more. The key is to guide your child, rather than to control his or her eating.

HOW TO EAT

Taking tension, pressure or haste out of eating can help to regulate your child's appetite, balance the amount they eat and ensure that their nutritional needs are met.

Children respond well to routine, and having regular meals is important for several reasons. First, a regular intake of food maintains energy levels in the body, which means they are less likely to snack on sugary, fatty foods. Second, it keeps your metabolism working, so you burn more calories faster. Third, it instils the idea that there are set times for eating, which can reduce the propensity to eat out of boredom or upset. It's fine to have some snacks between meals, of course, but try to limit these to a couple a day (toddlers may need more) and avoid giving snacks shortly before a meal.

EATING AS A FAMILY

Shared meals are a daily opportunity to promote good eating. Repeated studies show that children who participate in regular family meals are more likely to be a healthy weight. They also tend to eat more healthy foods, and to have improved psychological well-being.

Researchers can't say for sure that eating together is entirely responsible for such positive effects, because families that make time for shared meals may also engage in other practices that support well-being. However, a review of the evidence by researchers at Cornell University

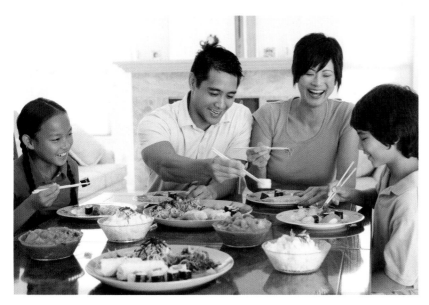

Eating together as a family as often as possible helps to promote a sense of belonging and stability as well as instilling children with good eating habits and manners – provided, that is, you offer healthy rather than junk food.

Try to encourage everyone to sit at a table to eat, rather than slumped on the sofa in front of the TV with a bowl of food. This not only promotes better digestion but also means you focus more on what you are eating and respond to satiety signals, helping to prevent overeating. It is also more sociable.

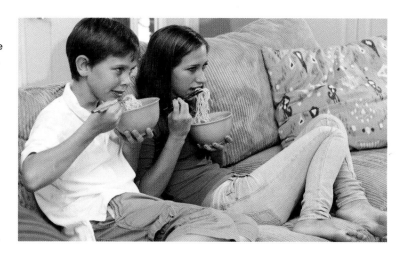

concluded that communal meals can play a significant part in generating a feeling of comfort and stability among family members, and in supporting healthy eating. Research has also shown that people tend to have more balanced meals and a greater variety of food when they eat with friends or family; your child can learn by seeing you make healthy choices.

The evidence suggests that sharing meals frequently provides the most benefits, so try to eat together at least three times a week. Getting together for a meal isn't always easy, especially when children are doing extracurricular activities and parents work or have their own activities. If so, be flexible about when and where you eat. Perhaps you could share your children's snack before bedtime? Make a point of having breakfast together? Have a picnic in the park? Or take the time for a weekend brunch? If older children or teens are reluctant, perhaps they would be keener if a friend were invited. And if there really seems no time, then look at the activities everyone is taking part in, and see what can be adjusted to make space for family time. It really is that important.

QUALITY AS WELL AS QUANTITY

Mealtimes should be pleasurable. Make time for them by putting away phones, turning off the TV, keeping toys off the table and family pets out of the room; these distractions can make adults and children alike much less likely to notice when they are full. Meals provide time to share thoughts, feelings and ideas – they are a key time for children to communicate with their parents. So try to keep mealtimes positive and stress-free. This is not the time to quiz your kids about bad behaviour and the like. But don't worry if the odd spat occurs – this is a normal part of family life for most of us.

It's very important to avoid battling over food with your children. If your child doesn't like the meal on offer, don't get drawn into an argument, which is both stressful and rarely achieves good results. Offering food without comment and then removing it, however much is left, within 20–30 minutes is often a wise approach. Whether eating together or not, encourage eating at the table, rather than on the sofa or in front of the TV. This helps your child to attend to their food, and sitting upright is better for digestion.

CHILDREN AND APPETITE

The amount a child eats may vary from day to day, and some kids want to eat more than others. Learning more about appetite can help you to ensure that your child is consuming a healthy quantity.

Many parents notice that one child in the family has a greater need for food than another, or seems more excited by the prospect of confectionery or other foods than their siblings. Scientists are discovering that there is a genetic element to appetite, and that this has an impact on weight gain. One study focused on non-identical three-month-old twin babies who had differing levels of two key aspects to appetite: food responsiveness (the urge to eat upon seeing or smelling food); and satiety responsiveness (the urge to stop eating when feeling full). Since the babies were the same age and sex, and growing up in the same family, any difference between them is probably genetic.

The study found that the twins who demonstrated lower fullness responsiveness or higher food responsiveness ate more, and put on more weight by the age of 15 months. The researchers suggested these children had a greater risk of becoming overweight or obese in the future than their twin, and that parents should be aware that a heartier appetite may go hand in hand with a tendency to overeat.

WHAT CAN PARENTS DO?
All children should be encouraged to notice when they are full, but children with a lower sensitivity to the internal signals of fullness will need particular help with this. Simply eating at a table and removing distractions such as the TV can help children to become more aware of the

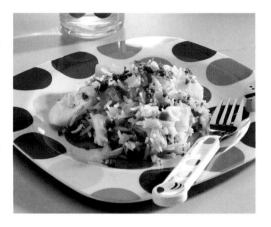

Use child-sized crockery and cutlery; not only will the portion size be appropriate, but it is more visually attractive for children.

sensation of fullness. Encourage your children to eat slowly and chew properly before swallowing. Don't persuade a young child to have a few more spoonfuls of a meal, or to clear the plate – this is teaching them to ignore their feelings of fullness and keep eating.

Some researchers have found that children who are allowed to serve themselves tend to eat the amount they need, rather than overeat. But serving food directly on to plates rather than putting serving dishes on the table may be more helpful for children who have a strong responsivity to food; it is also a good idea to keep snack foods out of sight.

Always offer (or encourage children to take) small portions to start with – larger portions are known to encourage both adults and children to eat more than they need – and then let them ask for more if they are still hungry when they have finished the first serving. It is a good idea to discourage children from having a second helping until 20 minutes after eating, to allow the body's feelings of fullness to develop.

GET THE RIGHT PLATES

Something as simple as changing the size of the crockery on which you serve your children's food can have an astonishing effect on the amount they eat – in one study, children were randomly given a small or large bowl and asked how much cereal and milk they wanted. Children who were given the large bowl asked for 87 per cent more than those given the small bowl – a huge difference.

In another study, children ate almost 50 per cent more when using an adult dinner plate than they did when they used a plate that was half the size. So it may well be worth buying special child-sized crockery for your children, or serving their food on a tea plate rather than a dinner plate.

ARE THEY REALLY HUNGRY?

There are lots of reasons why children may want to eat, apart from when they are actually hungry, such as boredom, emotional upset or habit. They may also find it difficult to distinguish between thirst and hunger. Next time your children say they are hungry, offer them some water to drink and distract them with an activity to keep them busy. The same applies for adults, too – instead of reaching for a cookie, have a glass of water. It will fill up your tummy and hydrate you at the same time.

HEALTHY EATERS
There are three key things that every healthy eater knows:

1 They know when they are hungry – and when they are not.

2 They are aware when they are eating – and how much.

3 They know when they are full – and stop!

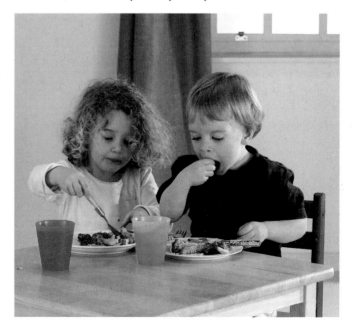

Give children small portions of food to start with, and allow them time to digest it before asking them if they want more.

SETTING FAMILY FOOD GOALS

There's no need to alter everything about your family's diet all at once – radical changes are hard to keep up. Small everyday changes will be less of a shock and much easier to stick to.

Most of us can improve our diet in some way – and if any members of the family are overweight, this is almost certainly the case. Ideally, change your family's eating habits gradually – a drastic overhaul is probably not going to be welcomed. That way, you are more likely to adopt a better diet permanently.

Change is much easier if everyone sees the reason for it, so speak to your children about the benefits of healthy eating. Talk in terms of feeling more energetic, doing better on the sportsfield (or being less out of breath when you walk) or having brainpower – rather than focusing on weight loss or reducing the risk of ill health. Preteens and teens, especially girls, may find the idea of clear skin, shiny hair and strong nails particularly compelling, while sporty kids may like the idea of building strong muscles. Ask your children to come up with some pros of healthy eating – you may find that they know more than you think.

If possible, agree some changes that you can all make. Your children may be good at coming up with ideas if challenged, or you may have to make the suggestions.

KEEPING A FOOD DIARY
It can help to keep a food diary for each member of the family. This can be a powerful tool that makes you aware of what foods you are all eating. You can scan or photocopy the blank one on page 154, or use an online one.

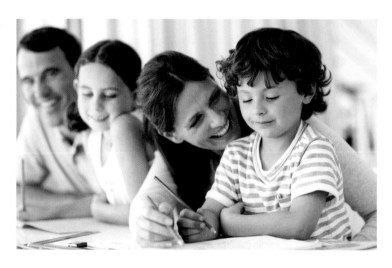

Sit down as a family to discuss and plan your goals before you start a new regime.

WHEN TO SEEK HELP
If you find it hard to make changes to your diet, your doctor may refer you to a dietician for practical advice and help. You should also discuss dietary changes with your doctor if your child is very overweight/obese or has health problems.

Right: Wholegrain cereals served with fruit make a nutritious and satisfying start to the day. Allowing children to help create some granola is a good way to encourage them to eat it.

Far right: A home-made muffin and some milk is a better snack option than processed food.

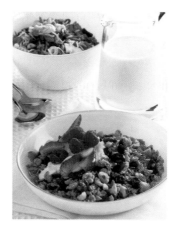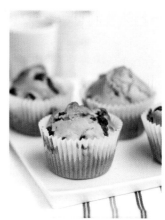

WHAT'S YOUR GOAL?

Every family's goals will be different, but here are some ideas that might work for you:

• Have wholemeal or whole-wheat bread or brown rice instead of white.
• Eat two vegetables or salad items with dinner.
• Add at least one salad vegetable to a packed lunch.
• Drink water with meals instead of soda.
• Cut out sugar in hot drinks.
• Switch sugary cereals for wholegrain cereals and a piece of fruit.
• Swap an after-school snack of crisps/potato chips or chocolate for a home-made muffin and a glass of milk.
• Serve smaller portions, and wait 20 minutes before having seconds or dessert.
• Share a sit-down family dinner several times a week.

It is best to fill in a food diary as you go through the day – it is all too easy to forget the odd cookie if you leave it until the evening. However, with schoolchildren, it is more practical to have set times for logging foods, such as after breakfast, after school and before bedtime – and to fill it in with them. Teenagers may be more motivated to complete an online food diary or to use an app on their phone.

Be sure to fill in everything that is consumed – for example, if you eat a ham salad at lunch, list the ingredients as 'tomatoes, lettuce, cucumber, grated carrot, slice of ham, mayonnaise' rather than simply 'salad'. Include drinks such as glasses of water or cups of tea (make a note of how many spoonfuls of sugar you add, if any). Try not to criticize any food choices your children record – it's important that everyone feels comfortable enough to be honest about what they are eating.

Keep it up for a week, then sit down as a family to look at the diaries. You may see at a glance that, say, your teenager is having soda every day at school, or that your family has got into the habit of having several takeaways a week without you really noticing. Or perhaps you will see that although you eat fairly healthily, you tend to have bigger portions than you need.

Talk it over, discuss your ideas and pick one or two goals to start with. It'll be easier to implement them if everyone agrees with the choice, or at least don't vehemently disagree with it. Go for the path of least resistance, while remaining committed to improving your family's diet choices.

PLANNING AND PREPARATION

Any lifestyle change needs a bit of planning. Here are the most effective ways to make your goals an integral part of your life.

When it comes to healthy eating, it's a good idea to remember that you are not aiming to be perfect, only better. Once you have decided on your goal, you need to set the date on which you are going to start. This gives everyone the chance to get used to the idea. So, if you have decided to have one dinner a week at the table with the TV off, take a look at your calendar and pick a good day. Write 'family meal' on the calendar. If your goal is to eat a healthier, wholegrain breakfast, decide when you are going to start. Choose a time when there isn't anything else going on, such as a sleepover with friends, a celebration or a holiday.

GET READY

Think about whether there is anything you need to do to get ready for the change. If your children are in the habit of eating packet cereals, for example, then you may want to finish what is already in the cupboard or pantry before you make the switch. Go shopping for some healthier alternatives, such as porridge

Preparing for a healthier way of living includes clearing out the cupboards and stocking up on nutritious fresh foods.

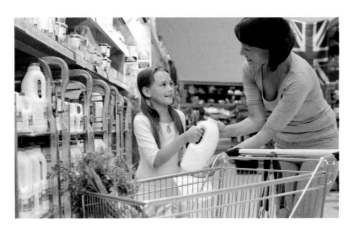

There are four stages to changing habits:

1 Contemplation – when you identify the change that is needed, consider how you are going to do it, and think about the pros and cons of changing your habits.

2 Preparation – this stage comes when you have made a decision that you want to change, and involves putting in place everything you will need to actually do it.

3 Action – this is when you are making the changes required to achieve your goal, overcoming obstacles, and adjusting to how it feels to act differently.

4 Maintenance – this final stage is when you have kept your change going, even if you have had set-backs and failings, and it now feels like a normal part of everyday life.

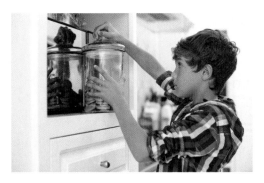

It is really important to clear the kitchen of jars of cookies and other unhealthy temptations.

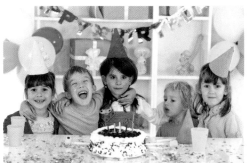

It is OK to relax the rules for special occasions, such as a party; enjoy it, then return to a healthy diet.

oats, wholewheat biscuit cereal or wholewheat bread, and the like. And think about whether there is something fun you can do to make the change appealing – perhaps new breakfast bowls for the kids?

GET STEADY

If you have picked a simple goal and the family resists, then you may have to drive through the change. Keep calm, sympathize with their complaints and reiterate that you all want to be healthier. Remember that you are an authority in the home – and sometimes you need to stand firm. It's more difficult if your partner is resistant; try to explain why the goal is a good idea. Make sure you remove temptation from the home – if your usual treats aren't in the kitchen, you can't eat them.

GO!

When the time comes to make the change, just do it. Be matter-of-fact: the decision has been made, the time is set. Photocopy and fill in the menu planner on page 155 and the family activity organizer on page 157 so that your kids know exactly what is expected and can tick off

the goals as they are met. This can give the whole family a sense of accomplishment. For extra motivation, think of a reward. One week of healthy breakfasts might result in a trip to your children's favourite park or leisure centre at the weekend, for example. Don't make the reward food-related.

MAINTENANCE

Eating healthily has to be a habit rather than a one-off activity, and you need to keep going. So add variety and plan new rewards. Don't worry if you slip up occasionally. It may help to have a 'don't miss twice' rule: missing your goal once is OK but twice in a row is not. Plan for special occasions, and allow your children to enjoy some of the healthier treats from the recipe section. Put a reminder on the calendar for the start of each week to stick to your goal.

Commit to 30 days: it takes this long for your goal to become a habit. Consider your next target – it may be much easier to get your family's agreement now that you have managed the first one, or you may be able to introduce a new healthier habit without them really noticing anything.

MENU PLANNERS

	BREAKFAST	SNACK OR DRINK
MONDAY	Berry and quinoa porridge (page 82)	Cheese straw (page 93) x 1 apple
TUESDAY	wholewheat biscuit cereal x 2 fresh berries	oatcakes x 2 banana
WEDNESDAY	Poached eggs on toast (page 86)	Mango and lime lassi (page 88) rice cakes
THURSDAY	wholemeal or whole-wheat toast with peanut butter orange	Hummus (page 90) with cucumber and celery sticks
FRIDAY	Granola and fruity topping (page 83) with yogurt	Artichoke and cumin dip (page 91) with celery sticks
SATURDAY	Dippy egg with toast soldiers (page 86)	Creamy banana boost (page 89) oatcake x 1
SUNDAY	Apple fritters (page 85) x 2	orange

LUNCH	**SNACK OR DRINK**	**DINNER**
Corn and potato chowder (page 104)	Raspberry smoothie (page 88)	Chicken casserole with vegetables (page 131)
Tortilla squares (page 110) carrot and cucumber sticks	Coconut berry popsicle (page 140) a handful of nuts	Fast fishes (page 126) with peas and salad
Chicken pasta salad (page 99) carrot sticks and tomatoes	Fruity flapjack (page 146) pear	Bulgur wheat with lamb (page 139) with green vegetables
Super-duper soup (page 103) with crusty bread	Banana muffin (page 149)	Spaghetti bolognese (page 138) with salad and green vegetables
Carrot soup (page 102) Cheese and potato bread twists (page 92)	apple	Fish kebabs (page 127) with brown rice and veg Rice pudding (page 144)
Crunchy veggie salad (page 108)	Fruity carrot cake (page 150)	Braised beans and lentils (page 125) with root-vegetable mash and greens
Braised beef with vegetables (page 137) Hedgerow crumble (page 145)	Peanut butter teabread (page 150)	Spudtastic with red bean chilli (pages 120–1) and salad

MENU PLANNERS

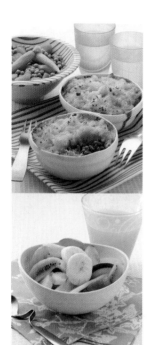

	BREAKFAST	SNACK OR DRINK
MONDAY	Ham and tomato scramble (page 87)	Almond and carrot bar (page 147)
TUESDAY	Granola and fruity topping (page 83) with yogurt	Cheese straw (page 93) apple or pear
WEDNESDAY	Berry and quinoa porridge (page 82)	Apricot bran muffin (page 84)
THURSDAY	Poached eggs on toast (page 86)	Artichoke and cumin dip (page 91) with carrot and cucumber sticks
FRIDAY	wholewheat biscuit cereal x 2 apple	Low-fat brownie (page 151)
SATURDAY	Buttermilk pancakes (page 85) raspberries or strawberries	Banana and mango thickie (page 89) oatcake x 1
SUNDAY	Dippy egg with toast soldiers (page 86)	pear rice cakes

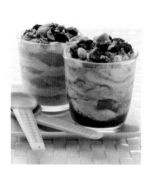

LUNCH	SNACK OR DRINK	DINNER
Lentil soup (page 104) with wholemeal or whole-wheat bread	Fabulous fruit salad (page 142)	Pan-fried chicken with pesto (page 130) with pasta and vegetables
Lemony couscous salad (page 100)	Date and muesli slice (page 146)	Roasted fish (page 127) with baked potato and broccoli
Roast tomato pasta salad (page 98)	Peanut dip (page 91) with vegetable strips	Tomato and lentil dhal (page 124) with brown rice and vegetables
Confetti salad (page 101) with tuna	Orange and apple rockie (page 148)	Tantalizing turkey burgers (page 132) with potato wedges, peas and corn
Chicken pitta pockets (page 94)	apple	Easy as fish pie (page 129) with vegetables
		Strawberry delight (page 142)
Popeye's pie (page 114) with salad	Carrot dip (page 90) with breadsticks	Bashed turkey with lime (page 133) with rice and vegetables
Super-duper soup (page 103) with wholemeal or whole-wheat bread	blueberries or grapes	Cottage pie (page 136) with carrots and peas
		Fruit fondue (page 143)

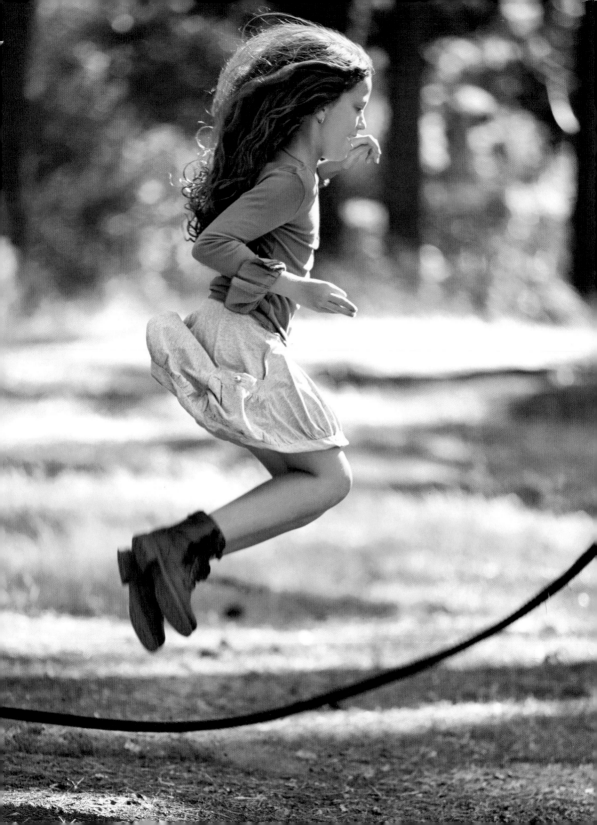

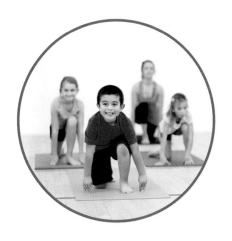

GETTING ACTIVE

In conjunction with good eating habits, exercise plays a vital role when it comes to achieving a healthy weight. This section explores how and why exercise is so good for us, and provides loads of inspiring ideas to get all the family moving, along with easy-to-use exercise planners and fun step-by-step routines.

WHY ACTIVITY MATTERS

Some children love being active; others need encouraging. Whether yours are natural athletes or cosy homebodies, they all need to get up and move.

Children need more exercise than adults – at least 60 minutes a day for those over five, and 180 minutes for the under-fives. Physical activity does more than burn calories: it builds strong bones and muscles, promotes self-confidence, and is also how children discover how their bodies work and how to solve problems.

Any form of physical activity and play counts as exercise. Ordinary childhood fun – swinging on the monkey bars, climbing a tree, skipping with a rope, playing tag – is fantastic exercise, and every few minutes counts towards the 60 a day (it doesn't have to be done in one go). Even so, the majority of children aren't active enough – one American study found that three out of four children over the age of five weren't exercising for the recommended 60 minutes per day. Less than 30 per cent of British children do sufficient exercise.

Swimming is a great way to strengthen muscles and burn off calories.

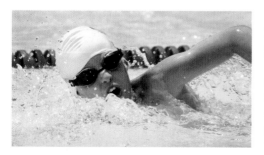

Part of the reason for this is that modern children have a lot less freedom than previous generations had. Over the past 20 years, the time children spend outdoors has dropped dramatically – a 2013 UK survey of 2,000 parents found that children spent half the time outdoors that their parents did, while an American study found that the average child was outside for just half an hour each day.

There are fewer opportunities for movement and exercise indoors, so children don't get the same chance to burn calories, and this means their physical abilities suffer. One UK study compared the strength of several hundred children with that of youngsters a decade earlier and found that the number of children who couldn't hold their own weight when hanging from the wall bars had doubled, while the number of sit-ups the children could do had dropped by more than 25 per cent. Even their ability to grip things with their hands had diminished.

WHAT KIND OF EXERCISE?
Children under the age of five should spend as little time as possible sitting down; they need to play and move around for three hours a day. Older children should do some sort of aerobic activity every day. Vigorous, bone-strengthening and muscle-strengthening activities should be done at least three times a week – some activities, including playing 'it', fulfil several criteria, so this isn't as complicated as it sounds.

BENEFITS OF EXERCISE

As well as helping to maintain a healthy weight, exercise:

- Increases muscle strength and endurance.
- Builds strong bones.
- Helps with general flexibility and balance.
- Promotes aerobic fitness.
- Gives a sense of well-being.
- Aids and enhances academic achievement.
- Enhances sleep.
- Improves hand-to-eye coordination and overall motor skills.
- Makes daily activities easier.

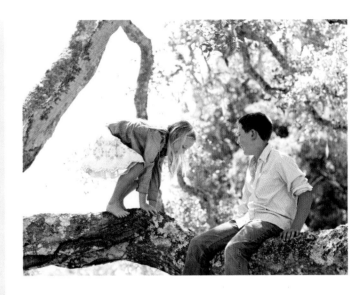

One UK survey (2011) found that a third of children had never climbed a tree, and one in ten had never ridden a bike.

Moderate activity

This includes activities that are physical enough to raise your heartbeat and increase your breathing. As a rule of thumb, you can probably talk while you do it, but not sing:
- walking to the stores or to school
- riding a scooter
- rollerskating or skateboarding
- cycling at a moderate pace
- using playground equipment

Vigorous activity

This is more intense exercise, making you breathe much harder and faster than normal, so you can't speak while doing it:
- disco, tap or other energetic dancing
- skipping with a rope
- running or playing 'it'
- team sports, such as netball, football etc
- fast or uphill cycling

Muscle-strength activity

This involves lifting your own body weight or working against resistance. (Generally, it is best for pre-pubescent children to avoid using weights, and older children should always be supervised and be sufficiently developed.)
- gymnastics
- modified press-ups or sit-ups
- climbing (indoor, rope, tree)
- swinging on playground equipment, such as monkey bars

Bone-strength activity

Any activity that creates impact or tension on the bones, which helps build strong bones:
- hopping, skipping or jumping
- skipping with a rope
- trampolining
- running
- gymnastics

THE PSYCHOLOGY OF EXERCISE

Children are primed to move – this is how babies explore their environment and develop their neural pathways. But little by little, many children lose interest in physical activity, or they simply drop the habit of movement from their daily routine.

Children who aren't naturally adept at physical activity may quickly realize it, especially once they start school. It's not uncommon for children as young as five to announce that they are 'no good' at sport once they start to compare themselves with their peers. This matters, because research shows that children who feel they are good at sport and who enjoy it are much more likely to take part in it. Children who see themselves as performing poorly are – not surprisingly – more likely to avoid sports.

If your children do not see themselves as sporty and are self-conscious or anxious about taking part in sports, there is a lot you can do to help them access their inner sports star – the part of them that wants to move, and take pleasure in their own physical potential.

FINDING THE SPORTS STAR WITHIN

Parental encouragement can be an important factor in the amount of exercise that children do. Here are seven ways you can help your child develop a more sport-friendly attitude:

1 Encourage them to know that exercise is for everyone – they just need to find what suits them. If they don't like team sports, no problem: they might like to try circus skills. Be positive about them trying out new forms of activity.

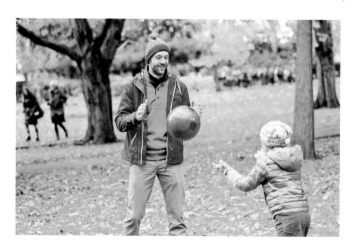

Play with your children! Getting out and about, playing catch or kicking a ball around not only improves their coordination, gets them moving and is great for bonding, but it also shows them that exercise is both a fun and a normal everyday activity.

2 Praise your child for having a go ('It's brilliant that you are trying out football') and for small achievements ('Hey, you walked much faster than last week'; 'See if you can do another length – but breaststroke this time'). One day at a time, you can help to build your child's sense of accomplishment.

3 Practice makes competent. Help your child learn the basic skills they use in school sports at home, out of sight of their peers and in a safe, non-judgemental environment. Playing catch, shooting a ball into a basket and kicking a football around will help your child improve without feeling too self-conscious. It can be a good idea to arrange one-on-one coaching for older children if they are really keen.

4 Pair them up. Children are often more willing to try something if they have a friend along – especially one who is similar in terms of ability. Offer your child the chance to learn to roller-skate with a friend, for example, or to join the same swimming class. Keep the emphasis on fun rather than winning or competition.

5 Have a go with them. A 10-minute game of catch or a kick-about is a wonderful way to have fun with your child. Learn something together, such as ice skating or hula-hooping – or train together for a fun run. It's good to let your child see you persevere with something that you are not naturally good at, so don't worry if it is hard for you to get the hang of it.

6 Be sure to let them know that you exercise. Children are much more likely to follow suit if they see their parents doing it. If you exercise when your children are at school, let them know about your fitness regime.

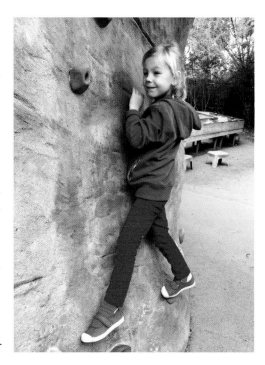

If your child doesn't like mainstream sports, try something different, such as climbing, circus skills, a martial art or yoga.

7 Notice your reactions. If your child is uncoordinated or out of shape, you may catch yourself feeling embarrassed or impatient when they can't do something. However, instead of commenting on the negative, make yourself notice something positive about what he or she is doing. Your child may not touch the ball in a football game, but do you notice he or she is defending well? It's very easy to buy into the idea that your child is 'no good' at sports – or to compare them with a more able friend or sibling – but you may miss some real achievements because of this and your negative attitude is not going to help their confidence.

WAYS TO GET ACTIVE

We tend to think of exercise as being organized sports – a football club, dance classes and the like. But there are lots of other ways of keeping fit without being the top scorer in the league.

When it comes to exercise for children, the basic rule is anything goes. The key thing is to make it fun, and make it regular.

All activity is exercise – children don't need to be doing sit-ups and press-ups to be working out. In fact, lots of adult forms of exercise aren't suitable for children, either because they are boring (running on a treadmill) or could be harmful (working out with heavy weights).

WALK IT
The simplest, most inexpensive way to get your child fitter is to ditch the car and walk where you need to go. If you can walk to school each

A family walk in the park or countryside is a great, free weekend or after-school activity.

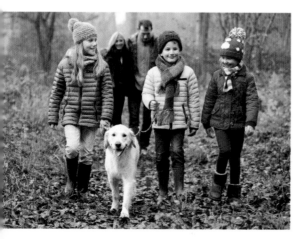

day, great. If not, schedule in a regular trip to the local store, library or similar. Take small opportunities to increase your child's activity: park the car 10 minutes away from where you want to get to; take the stairs rather than the elevator or escalator; when dinner is over, go for a walk round your neighbourhood rather than slumping in front of the TV. Walking with your child gives you a chance to chat that you may not otherwise get – enjoy it.

SCOOT WITH YOUNG ONES
Younger children tire easily, and it can be incredibly frustrating to walk with them when you are in a hurry to get somewhere for a set time. A three-wheeled scooter makes it more fun for them – and much quicker for you. Get them used to wearing a helmet: even two-year-olds can be pretty speedy on a scooter, and their heads need to be protected in case they fall off. Make sure they understand and obey rules about roads and stop when you tell them to.

HAVE ACTIVE PLAYDATES
When your children have friends over, insist that they play a game rather than turn on the TV or check their tablets. Take them to the park to play tag, throw a frisbee or kick a ball, go swimming, or get them playing in the garden. If it is wet, let them play hide-and-seek (you can lay down a few ground rules, if you like, such as banning them from your bedroom).

THE GAME OF SEVENS

All you need for this game is a bouncy ball and an expanse of wall. You throw the ball in different ways, a set number of times each go, without dropping it. If you drop the ball, then it's your competitor's turn; you have to start at the same number when it is your turn again. Or, if you are playing on your own, just start the round again.

7 Throw the ball against the wall, then catch it before it hits the ground. Do this seven times.

6 Throw the ball, let it bounce on the ground, then catch it. Do this six times.

5 Drop the ball on the ground and use the palm of your hand to make it bounce five times.

4 Lift one leg, throw the ball under it and against the wall, then catch it. Do this four times.

3 Throw the ball against the wall, let it drop on the ground and use the palm of your hand to make it bounce three times. Do this three times.

2 Throw the ball against the wall, then quickly clap your hands together in front of you, behind you and in front of you once more, before catching it. Do this twice.

1 Throw the ball against the wall, spin round on one foot (in a 360-degree circle) and catch the ball before it drops to the ground. Do this once.

Once you have completed all seven rounds, you can do it again, but this time you are not allowed to move to catch the ball but must stay on the same spot. The next variation is to do the seven rounds one-handed – expert level!

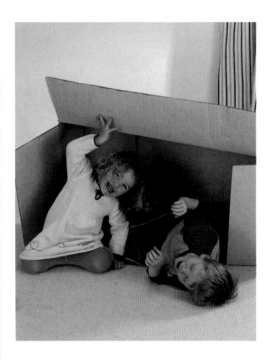

Be imaginative when it comes to playdates – an old box makes a perfect hiding place or den.

BUILD A DEN

This can be a great way to get your child moving and stretching without even realizing they are exercising. Get some materials together – a plastic sheet or old cloth, string, bamboo canes, pegs (pins), a few boxes of different sizes – and let the children choose which ones to use. If you are outside, set the children to collect old fallen branches to supplement your materials. If you are inside, they can incorporate tables, chairs and other furniture. It's a good idea to show your children how to tie knots or use pegs to keep the sheet up – but often they will have strong ideas about what they want to build. Younger children may also like to build mini–dens for their toys.

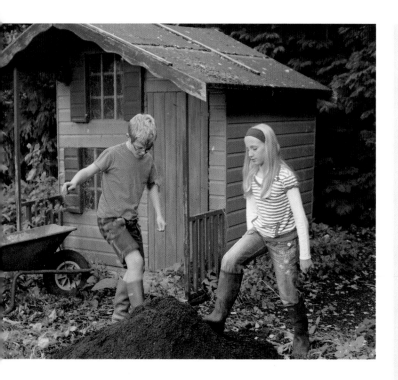

Here are three good moves to try out on the trampoline:

1 Star jumps – as you jump, spread your arms and legs wide to make a star shape. Bring them back together in time for your landing.

2 High knees – bring your knees towards your chest and touch your feet, before bringing them back down into the usual jump position.

3 Butt drops – bring your legs out in front of you after you jump, so that you land and bounce in a seated position. As you come back up, bring your legs back to standing for the next jump.

Gardening is very good exercise, and most children enjoy getting involved. Just ensure they wear appropriate footwear and clothing.

GET OUT IN THE GARDEN

Even a tiny garden can be turned into a mini-sports arena. Get a couple of hula hoops, a basketball hoop, a pogo stick, a couple of rackets and a soft ball, or teach your child the game of sevens (page 49). Keep some outdoor toys packed away so you can produce them when your children are bored. Children also love helping to garden, so enlist their help with digging, sowing, pruning and harvesting.

GET A TRAMPOLINE

If you have space, then a trampoline is a fantastic addition to the garden. Trampolining is a highly effective way to keep fit – a 10-minute session provides the same health benefits as a 30-minute run, and it is one of the best ways to improve coordination. It's also non-intimidating – even the most sports-averse child is likely to have a go. Do make sure that you buy a good-quality trampoline with a safety net and padding, and supervise your children to ensure that only one child at a time uses it. They should bounce in the middle, and not attempt gymnastic-style tricks. Under-sixes should use a trampoline designed for young children.

PLAY PARK OLYMPICS

Make a point of visiting your local park, even for a few minutes, after school and at weekends.

Challenge your kids to play park olympics – in which you race to use each piece of apparatus: hand-walk the monkey bars, go down each slide, swing on every swing. Use a stopwatch to see how fast they can get round the park.

EMBRACE THE SEASONS

Get outside with your children whatever the weather: wrap up warm and go sledging or have a snowball battle when it snows; catch falling leaves in autumn; splash in puddles; fly a kite on windy days. After a while, it will become second nature to be out and about.

GET ON YOUR BIKE

Cycling is fantastic cardiovascular exercise, and it's easy to fit into your day if you use it as a form of transport. It's low-impact, so it is gentle on the joints, but builds muscle in the legs and buttocks. And if you ride off-road or in the hills it increases upper-body strength too. If possible, let your children cycle to school – one study of almost 20,000 Danish children found that those who cycled or walked to school did much better at tasks involving concentration when they got there and for up to four hours afterwards. Otherwise, go for family rides at the weekend, or as often as possible.

TEAM UP

At the weekends, meet up with other families to do something active. Invest in a set of boules – French bowling balls – or a croquet set. Play rounders, cricket, volleyball or football together. Or head for the hills and go for a long cycle ride or hike. It's much easier to get your children involved and enthusiastic if there are other children around, and this sort of multi-family event can be a good way to engage teenagers too.

HOLD A TOURNAMENT

Go to your local pound/dollar store and pick up a selection of prizes – stickers, stationery, silly hats and the like. Then challenge your children to a tournament, held in your garden or the local park. Give prizes for the fastest running-on-the-spot, the most elegant set of star jumps (jumping jacks), or the funniest way of getting from A to B – or anything else you can think of. Be sure to choose competitions your children can actually manage, and to spread the prize-winning reasonably evenly so that nobody gets upset or feels like a failure.

GO JUGGLE

Get a set of juggling balls – it's an enjoyable activity, and it is as good an exercise as walking, with lots of arm movements and plenty of squats as you bend to pick up the balls. It is also great for developing hand-to-eye coordination. If your children find it hard to get the hang of the technique, get them to try with lightweight juggling scarves (readily available online). Look online for some useful videos on technique.

Whatever the weather, invite over your children's friends and encourage them to play outside.

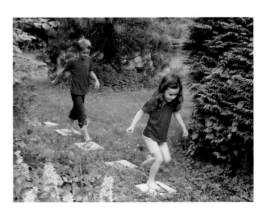

HOW TO PLAY HOPSCOTCH

Draw the hopscotch squares on the ground, using chalk. Make each square large enough for someone to hop into – square 10 should be large enough for you to be able to turn round, and 3/4 and 6/7 should be double squares, as shown below.

1 Throw a flat pebble or small non-breakable object on to the first square – it has to go inside the lines (you lose your go if it lands on a line).

2 Hop from one square to the next, avoiding the one that holds your pebble, and keeping your foot inside each square (no treading on the lines). When you get to the end, turn around (remaining on one foot), and then retrace your steps.

3 When you get to the square before the one holding your marker, bend down (on one foot), pick it up and then hop to your starting point (outside the hopscotch design). Then throw the marker on to square 2, and repeat as above.

4 Your go ends when you lose your balance, tread on the lines, or do not throw your marker into the right square. Once you reach square 10, you are the winner.

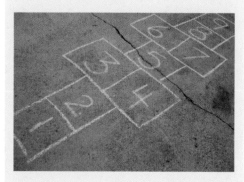

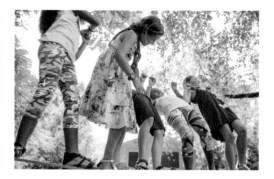

A slackline is great fun to use. Younger children may need a hand rope to help them get across.

WALK THE ROPE

Introduce your children to a slackline – a wide tightrope quite low to the ground, similar in thickness to a seatbelt, which is anchored between two points. It's a great way to work on balance and helps promote physical confidence. You'll need to supervize your child and read the safety instructions carefully. If you are using one between two trees, be sure to get tree protectors.

INVEST IN PEDOMETERS

Everyone loves a gadget. A pedometer can be a great way to encourage your child to walk more. Give your child lots of small targets to reach – how many steps to the end of the road or how quickly can you take 50 steps? Get a pedometer for every member of the household, and compare how many steps you take each day – healthy competition can be a great motivator.

ARRANGE A CLASS

Sports such as basketball, football etc are fantastic for fitness, but there are plenty of other activities for children to enjoy if they are not team players. Ask your child what they want to try – indoor climbing, table tennis, martial arts.

Most teachers will let you try out a class before you sign up. Keep going until you find something your child likes. Many are influenced by what is fashionable; a modern dance class that uses current music may be a lot more appealing than classical ballet. Or your child might like to try street dance, skateboarding or capoeira.

TURN A WALK INTO AN ADVENTURE

Enthuse even the most reluctant walker by turning your walk into a voyage of discovery. Make a list of 10 things you want your children to spot in the neighbourhood – a postbox, a red car, a black dog, a man wearing a hat. This is a brilliant way of making a nature walk seem more appealing – 'find me a pine cone', 'look for three different types of leaf', and so on. Or try giving each child a tray filled with a layer of soil, then tell them you are going out to find items to turn their tray into a magical garden. Look for pebbles, leaves, twigs, shells and other small things that they can use. Supplement these with household items – string, foil and the like.

HAVE A TREASURE HUNT

Younger children – and quite a few older ones – love treasure hunts, and this can be a novel way to entice them off the couch. Spend a few minutes writing some clues that will lead your children around the local neighbourhood – they should lead the finder from one landmark to the next. Hide each clue and watch your children race from one to the next. Make the prize a non-food item, such as stickers or toys.

INDOORS

If you are stuck indoors, try creating a mini obstacle course to get your kids moving. Be creative about what you use: small sturdy items of furniture, hula hoops, bean bags, footballs and soft toys can all work well. Once you have set up an obstacle course, your kids might want to take over and set up their own – get them to do one for you, and then show you how to use it.

TUNE IN, GET DOWN

Simply ramp up the music and dance. Games consoles can also be a real boon here – there are plenty of dance and sports games that keep your children amused and on their feet. Online, there are loads of workout or dance videos that you can make use of. Do count this as part of their screentime, though.

HOUSEHOLD CHORES

Not everyone's idea of fun, granted, but helping at home can be a good way to increase your child's activity rate. Washing the windows or the car involves lots of stretching, and dusting, vacuuming or weeding the garden can provide a decent workout if you do it with some energy. Even laying the table or emptying the dishwasher involves movement. And by helping out, your children should save you a little time, which you can use to play with them.

By committing to, and paying for, a regular class, you are more likely to stick with a routine.

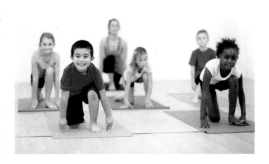

SENSIBLE SCREENTIME

Today's parents face a challenge that no previous generation before them has had to deal with – how to limit their children's screentime. It's easy to let the hours slip, but spending too long in front of a screen affects a child's weight and well-being.

More than 25 years ago, researchers noted a correlation between watching a lot of television and weight gain. Since then a host of studies has confirmed that excessive TV-watching is linked to obesity and weight gain – and that the effects last well into adulthood.

Is TV really so bad for our children? Well, yes it is, when they watch it for hours. When they sit down, they are inactive – and the more time that is spent in front of the TV, the less there is available for more energetic pursuits. In addition, watching TV encourages a taste for the kinds of high-calorie, low-nutrient foods that are linked to weight gain, because of the advertisements and product placements that are strategically aired between programmes.

One study found that children watching cartoons interspersed with advertisements for food ate substantially more snacks than those watching non-food commercials. Overweight and obese children had the largest increase in their calorie intake. Another five-year study found that the more hours of commercial TV children watched, the greater the likelihood of an increase in their BMI at the end of the study. To make things worse, there are other negative effects. The light from TVs (and computer monitors) can interfere with the natural body clock and impede sleep, a lack of which is also associated with weight gain (see pages 56–7).

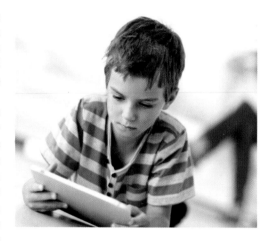

Screentime is not just restricted to watching TV; using tablets, smartphones, games consoles and computers all count and need to be limited.

Of course, today's children don't just watch TV; they also have games consoles, tablets, smartphones and computers. These are more interactive than watching TV, and the link between using them and excess weight gain is less clear – some studies have found a connection, others have not. Even so, most kinds of screentime cause children to sit and seem to encourage snacking. So it makes sense to reduce screentime as a whole rather than to concentrate on TV-watching alone.

REDUCING SCREENTIME

The American Academy of Pediatrics recommends that children over the age of three (including teenagers) should have no more than two hours of quality screentime a day. Children aged under three shouldn't have any screentime at all; their brains are developing rapidly at this age, and they need plenty of human interaction and playtime. Here is how to cut down:

Unplug bedrooms Keep TVs and other electronics out of children's bedrooms – research shows that having a TV in the bedroom is linked to weight gain. It's also easier to monitor what your children are watching if the TV is in a communal area

Silence the smartphones Have a family rule that phones are to be placed on a shelf for certain periods during the day, rather than being kept constantly to hand. Don't allow phones in the bedroom.

Lead by example As your children's main role model, you need to ensure that your screentime is under control, too. Stick to the same rules, and don't constantly check or play on your phone when you are around your children. **Eat without screens** Don't have the television as background noise during mealtimes or when other activities (homework, playing etc) are taking place. This makes it harder for your child to concentrate. Use the time for conversation. **Make a schedule** Rather than banning the screen completely, agree a set limit to your children's screentime (see the activity and screentime diary on page 62). Involve them in deciding the schedule – they'll be less resistant if they have had a say (though they still shouldn't watch TV in the hour before bedtime). **Provide alternatives** Have a music player in the living room and in your children's bedrooms, so that they can put on some music and dance.

Most of us enjoy watching TV some of the time, and using a tablet or some form of computer is a normal part of everyday life. It can easily get out of hand, however, so it is really important to monitor and assess the amount of time your whole family is spending sitting down in front of a screen. You can then set limits together, and write them on a chart so that you can track your progress and see if you achieve your goals.

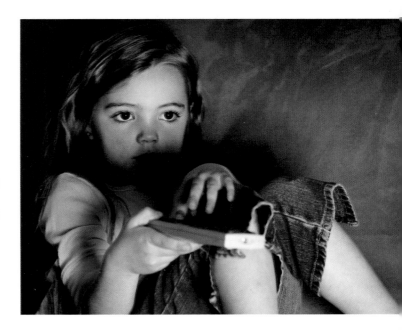

ALL ABOUT SLEEP

It's hard to eat sensibly or exercise when you are deprived of sleep. Making sure your child is getting enough rest is an important factor in helping them to maintain a healthy weight and stay well.

Various studies have suggested that poor sleep is associated with excess weight gain in children and adults. A British study tracking 8,000 children found that those who had fewer than 10½ hours' sleep a night at the age of three were 45 per cent more likely to be obese by the age of seven.

There are many reasons why poor sleep may impact on weight. When you are tired, sugary, high-fat snacks offer a tempting quick boost. Activity is also less appealing when you are feeling weary – while a lack of exercise can also lead to poorer sleep, creating a vicious circle. Lack of sleep also disrupts the balance of hormones in the body. People deprived of sleep tend to have low levels of leptin, a hormone that sends a message to the brain when the body has sufficient stores of fat. They also have higher-than-normal levels of the hormone ghrelin, the function of which is to trigger hunger pangs. The combined effect of such imbalances is a tendency to overeat.

HOW MUCH SLEEP DO CHILDREN NEED?

The American National Sleep Foundation recommends that children get the following amount of sleep:

Toddlers (1–3):
  12–14 hours
Preschoolers (3–5):
  11–13 hours
School-aged children (5–10):
  10–11 hours
High-school children (11–12):
  9–12 hours
Teenagers (13+): 10–12 hours

This is per 24-hour period, and includes any naps. On average, children get an hour less sleep than they should.

Teenagers in particular can really suffer from early starts after an insufficient amount of sleep, so make a sensible bedtime a priority and be firm about screentime, especially in the hour before they go to bed. Limit late-evening activities and insist on a consistent routine.

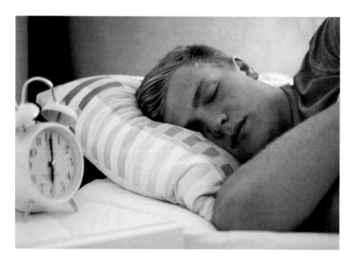

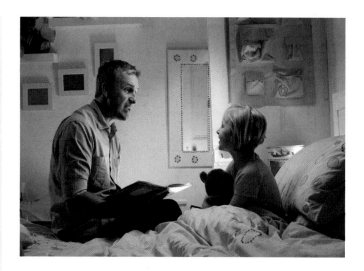

Make bedtime as relaxing as possible, with dim lighting, a clutter-free space and, for younger children, a soothing story.

And, of course, lack of sleep doesn't just impact on weight. If your child doesn't get enough sleep, he or she may be over-emotional, irritable, forgetful, may struggle to concentrate and could wake frequently in the night.

IMPROVING SLEEP

Be regular Going to bed and getting up at the same time each day helps to set the body clock. Try not to vary this time by more than an hour.
Go to bed early Going to bed after 9pm can result in your child taking longer to fall asleep and getting less sleep overall. Encourage as much homework as possible be done at weekends, to reduce the pressure on weeknights, and limit late-evening activities on school nights.
Have a sleeptime routine Doing the same calming activities each night before bedtime will help your child feel sleepier. Try a warm bath, followed by milk, teeth cleaning, and a story or gentle song. Avoid active play.

Make your child's bedroom comfortable Make it a pleasurable, clutter-free place to be. Keep the temperature at around 18.5°C (65°F), the optimal temperature for sleep.
Make it dark Children are sensitive to light, so use black-out blinds or thick curtains. Keep lights low during the bedtime routine, and switch off electronics that glow.
Monitor TV use Don't let your child watch scary programmes that may cause nightmares. Don't watch TV in the hour before bedtime.
Keep caffeinated drinks out of your child's diet Teas, coffees and colas contain stimulating caffeine, which impedes sleep.
Seek advice If your child gets less than the recommended number of hours asleep – or if he or she wakes up because of snoring – see your doctor. Many sleep conditions can be treated. Medications or conditions such as ADHD can impact on sleep, so need discussing with a medical professional.

SETTING GOALS

If you are committed to getting your children to be more active, the best way to achieve this is to have specific goals. Here is a way of clarifying what yours should be.

The first step when setting your family's activity goals is to ensure that you are aware of your current habits. So, for a week, make a note of how much exercise the adults and children in your household do. Print out the blank activity and screentime diary on page 156, or make your own, with a column for each member of the family, and two rows – one for activity and one for screentime. Get your kids involved right from the start by explaining that you are going to record how much you all do. If they are enthusiastic, they may want to fill in their own column. However, do be sure it is accurate.

Children will enjoy filling in their part of the chart, so get them involved right from the start.

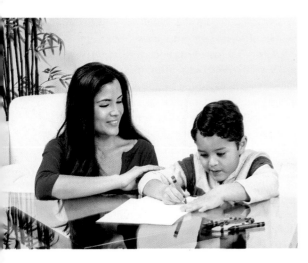

At the end of each day, tot up how much exercise each individual has done – your children may enjoy being a little competitive about this – and how much screentime they've had. Include time spent in front of the TV, video games, tablets and the computer.

Talk about the results with your children if they are old enough to understand. Explain that they should be aiming to be active for an hour a day at least, and that they should have no more than two hours of screentime (for most under-fives, you are better off distracting them from screentime with games rather than trying to convince them it's good for them not to watch TV). Share your feeling that you all need to be more active as a family, and that taking lots of little steps will help to make you all feel healthier in the long term.

HOW TO SET GOALS

Think about how you want to change your family's routine, and the goals you want to set. It is a good idea to enlist your children's help in setting some goals. Make sure that they are:

Realistic Accept the current situation. If your children are overweight and unused to exercise then it's not fair to expect them to, say, join a running club or a gymnastics class with children who have been doing it for years.

Achievable It's better to have a small, manageable goal that you can attain – that way, you'll feel good about yourselves and be more

Doing one of the workout routines outlined in the planner on pages 64–5 as a family is a very realistic and achievable goal, since all it requires is some comfortable clothing, a little time and some commitment. By doing it together you can boost each other's morale, inject a little healthy competition into the activity and, crucially, all get a bit fitter.

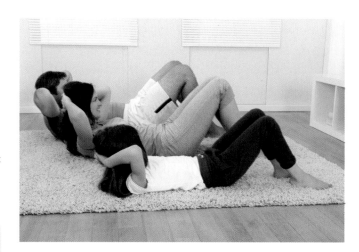

FAMILY GOALS

Here are a few ideas that might suit your family:

• Each child can choose an exercise or dance class to do one day after school or at the weekend.
• Everyone to walk to school or work at least once a week, preferably every day if at all possible. If it is too far away, agree to walk part of the way.
• The whole family to enjoy an active outing together every weekend.
• The whole family to participate in an activity – 10-pin bowling, ice skating, swimming, cycling, hiking.
• Nobody to spend more than two hours a day looking at a screen (excluding adults' work and any homework).
• Parent and child to train together for a fun walk or run.

likely to continue. If you set your sights too high, you may fail and give up on the idea of being healthier altogether. If your family is doing very little exercise, set yourselves the target of attending one exercise class a week rather than going running every day, for instance.

Specific 'We're going to be more active' is difficult to stick to; 'we are going to walk to school every morning' is much more concrete and deliverable, so be precise.

Each family's goals will be a little different. Remember that the emphasis should be on having fun with exercise – any weight loss and health benefits should really be viewed as a bonus. It's important that you all do something that you enjoy – you may love football, but if your children hate it then there is no point in pushing them to do it.

PLAN AHEAD

One of the best ways to regulate everybody's activities is to sit down as a family and fill in a family activity organizer (you can photocopy the one on page 157). That way you can accurately gauge whether everyone is doing sufficient exercise, and it also helps prevent arguments during the week, since you can just point to the organizer and show the exercise or activity that was agreed to. We have filled in the first day for a fictitious family as an example on page 63; now use the blank one on page 157 to map out your own family's week.

PLANNING AND PREPARATION

Sorting out everything you need in advance, and setting a specific date for when the new routine will start, means that everyone will be prepared and ready to adopt a healthier lifestyle.

Decide on a date when you are going to start your new regime – a week from today, perhaps, or further into the future if more planning is involved. If possible, agree the date together as a family; otherwise, make sure you let everyone know what has been decided well in advance.

Next, research what you need to know about your goals. If you have decided that each child is going to take a weekly class, for example, find out what is on offer. Ask other parents what their children are doing. Search online for details of local classes. Again, get your children involved – task everyone with coming up with a suggestion for a class they can join, or get them to write down two suggestions for a weekend family outing. Take care not to criticize any outlandish suggestions, but encourage everyone to write down some practical ideas as well as fantasies.

Make a list of the kit you need for your chosen activities, and buy or borrow anything you don't already have. Even if there is no uniform, your children may need new trainers or comfortable clothing they can stretch in. Find a place to store the kit – it is a good idea to keep it in a bag so everything is on hand when you need it. Work out the logistics. If your children want to do a class that is a few miles away, how will they get there? Can you facilitate what they want to do?

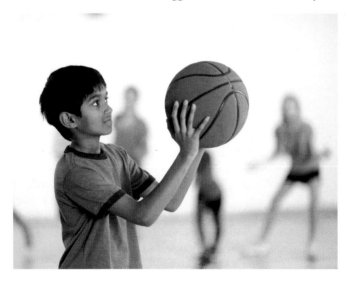

YOUR FOUR-POINT ACTION PLAN
1 Set a date.
2 Find out what you need to know.
3 Get what you need.
4 And you're off!

Getting your children to classes and activity sessions at the right time and wearing the correct clothing requires planning and preparation. A family activity organizer can help everybody know what is going on and when.

MY CHILDREN DON'T WANT TO DO IT!

Don't be deterred if your children seem resistant to the plans; people often dislike the idea of change, especially when it involves effort. Children are very good at coming up with reasons for not doing something. Be sympathetic but firm and don't change your plan. This is when you, the parent, needs to be an authority. It's helpful to think of exercise as an essential part of your family's routine – like using a car seat, or cleaning teeth.

A new routine may be more attractive to children if you create a reward system – just as you may have done a star chart to help with potty training or sleeping through the night. Depending on how resistant your children are, you might want to schedule a small reward at the end of the first week, or perhaps every half-term. Make sure the prize isn't something like ice cream or a takeaway pizza. An exercise-related incentive – such as new jogging trainers – would be great, but a book or small toy would work well, too. Make sure the reward is linked to effort (turning up to a class, say) rather than performance (getting selected to play for the school or scoring a goal).

SCHEDULE IT IN

It's helpful – in fact it's practically essential – to have a day-by-day family activity organizer (like the ones on page 63 and page 157) that shows the precise times of classes, school events and other activities. This allows you to see at a glance who is meant to be doing what on which day in terms of activity levels. As members of the family achieve their goals they can put a tick in the 'Tick?' column, which gives everybody a sense of satisfaction. Keep the charts you have filled in, so you can assess where things need adjusting.

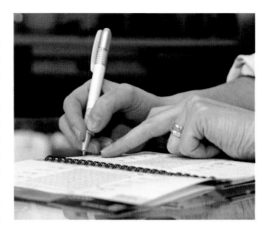

Filling in a planner is a great way to work out exactly what your aims are, and it serves as a written reminder whenever you look at it.

USING PLANNERS

The purpose of planners is to create a statement of intention for the week ahead when it comes to activities, workouts or menus. This enables you to get organized and think carefully about creating a balanced and healthy activity schedule, or plan meals in advance – rather than deciding what to do or eat on the spur of the moment.

We have carefully collated the workout and menu planners featured in this book, but you can easily create your own if you prefer. Just bear in mind that you are aiming for a good balance of stretches and cardio activities, and that all the food groups should be covered and the daily calorie intake should fall within the guidelines for each age group, as outlined on pages 14–15. You should also ensure that there is variety throughout the week. Planners are intended to be helpful tools, but they are also a record of an agreed strategy that can be referred to when resistance is encountered.

ACTIVITY AND SCREENTIME DIARY

	CHILD 1	CHILD 2	PARENT	PARENT
MONDAY Activity	• cycle to and from school (20 mins) • football (40 mins)	• walk to school (15 mins) • work out (30 mins)	• walk to school (15 mins) • work out (30 mins)	• cycle to and from work (40 mins)
Screentime	• TV (15 mins) • console (1 hour)	• surf internet (1 hour)	• internet shopping (15 mins)	• watch a film (2½ hours)
TUESDAY Activity				
Screentime				
WEDNESDAY Activity				
Screentime				
THURSDAY Activity				
Screentime				
FRIDAY Activity				
Screentime				
SATURDAY Activity				
Screentime				
SUNDAY Activity				
Screentime				

FAMILY ACTIVITY ORGANIZER

	WHAT	WHEN	WHO	TICK?
MONDAY	• walk to school • cycle to school and work • football • cycle home • workout 1	8.20am 8.20am 3.30pm 5pm 4pm–4.30pm	Clara and Mum Peter and Dad Peter Peter and Dad Clara and Mum	
TUESDAY				
WEDNESDAY				
THURSDAY				
FRIDAY				
SATURDAY				
SUNDAY				

WORKOUT ROUTINE PLANNER

BEFORE YOU BEGIN

These plans mix and match exercises from the four different sections that start overleaf. Read the workout advice for each before you start, and adapt exercises to your children's fitness and flexibility. Warm up for 5–6 minutes before doing more intense moves, and don't push your or your child's body further than it will naturally go.

WORKOUT 1

March like a soldier (page 66)
Shimmy to the side (page 67)
Run on the spot (page 68)
Bend to the side (page 68)
Shoulder stretch (page 69)
Star jumps (jumping jacks) (page 70)
The leg pendulum (page 70)
Pull-downs (page 71)
Toe kicks (page 72)
Frog jumps (page 73)
Curl-ups (page 74)
Downward dog (page 78)
Cat-to-cow pose (page 78)
Child's pose (page 79)

WORKOUT 2

Walk on the spot for 5 minutes
Hit your knee (page 68)
Kick your butt (page 68)
Punch the piñata (page 67)
Bend to the side (page 68)
Clocks and windmills (page 69)
Swing out (page 71)
Giant's steps (page 72)
Crab walking (page 73)
Mountain climbing (page 75)
Triceps dips (page 76)
Upward dog/cobra pose (page 79)
Bent-leg stretch (page 77)
Butterfly (page 79)

WORKOUT 3

Run on the spot (page 68)
Shimmy to the side (page 67)
Toe kicks (page 72)
Pull-downs (page 71)
The leg pendulum (page 70)
Walk like a creepy-crawly (page 71)
Frog jumps (page 73)
Seal walking (page 72)
Squats (page 74)
Hang loose (page 77)
The stork (page 77)
Giant stretch (page 77)
Lie down and breathe

WORKOUT 4

March like a soldier (page 66)
Punch the piñata (page 67)
Star jumps (jumping jacks) (page 70)
Swing out (page 71)
Run on the spot (page 68)
Aeroplane (page 69)
Hit your knee (page 68)
Kneeling push-ups (page 75)
Plank (page 76)
Seal walking (page 72)
Cat-to-cow pose (page 78)
Butterfly (page 79)
Bent-leg stretch (page 77)

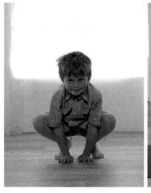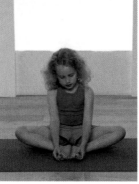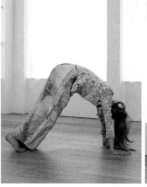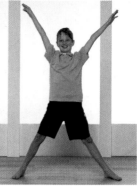

WORKOUT 5

Walk on the spot for 5 minutes
Run on the spot (page 68)
Bend to the side (page 68)
Kick your butt (page 68)
Shimmy to the side (page 67)
Punch the piñata (page 67)
Shoulder stretch (page 69)
Clocks and windmills (page 69)
The leg pendulum (page 70)
Giant's steps (page 72)
Burpee (page 76)
Downward dog (page 78)
Cat-to-cow pose (page 78)
Lie down and breathe

WORKOUT 6

Run on the spot (page 68)
Star jumps (jumping jacks) (page 70)
Kick your butt (page 68)
Squats (page 74)
Mountain climbing (page 75)
Swing out (page 71)
Curl-ups (page 74)
March like a soldier (page 66)
Plank (page 76)
Giant stretch (page 77)
Bent-leg stretch (page 77)
Hang loose (page 77)
Cat-to-cow pose (page 78)
Butterfly (page 79)

WORKOUT 7

Walk on the spot for 5 minutes
Kick your butt (page 68)
Toe kicks (page 72)
Kneeling push-ups (page 75)
Squats (page 74)
Curl-ups (page 74)
Pull-downs (page 71)
Triceps dips (page 76)
March like a soldier (page 66)
The stork (page 77)
Upward dog/cobra pose (page 79)
Downward dog (page 78)
Child's pose (page 79)

WORKOUT 8

Run on the spot (page 68)
Bend to the side (page 68)
Hit your knee (page 68)
Shoulder stretch (page 69)
Clocks and windmills (page 69)
Kick your butt (page 68)
Plank (page 76)
Star jumps (jumping jacks) (page 70)
Burpee (page 76)
Squats (page 74)
Seal walking (page 72)
Bent-leg stretch (page 77)
Lie down and breathe

WAKE UP, WARM UP

This is a brilliant set of exercises to do as a warm-up, or for a jump-around on a rainy day. It is good for all ages – from toddlers to adults.

When exercising with children, the thing that matters most is to keep it fun, fun, fun. Don't take it too seriously – exercise should never feel punishing or forced. If you are playful and enthusiastic, then your kids will be, too.

KEEP SAFE

These exercises are suitable for healthy children, but do take into account your child's individual strength and flexibility. If your child has health problems, is injured or is overweight, talk to your doctor first about an individually tailored exercise programme.

WORKOUT TIPS

• Plan which exercises you will do in advance.
• Keep home workouts short and snappy, and let your child go at their own pace. Do encourage, but never force.
• Wear trainers or go barefoot rather than wearing shoes. Put on stretchy comfortable clothing – leggings or shorts and a T-shirt.
• Have water to hand, and take breaks when you need to.
• Never continue with an exercise that hurts! Build up the reps and intensity gradually, respecting everyone's limits.

March like a soldier

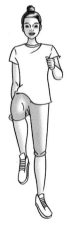 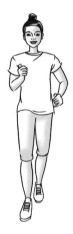 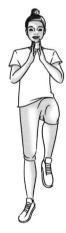

1 March on the spot. Pump your arms as you work the legs, keeping the fists soft. Count from one to eight – 'one, two, three, four, five, six, seven, eight' – as you march. Keep it going for 30 seconds.

2 Now march forwards four steps, counting out 'one, two, three, four', and clap your hands twice. Then march four steps back, counting 'hup, two, three, four', and clap your hands twice more.

3 Mid-march, stand on one leg as you clap for 30 seconds, then repeat 30 seconds of on-the-spot marching, and another 30 seconds of back-and-forth marching. Say 'hup, two, three, four' as you do it.

Shimmy to the side

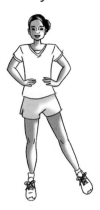
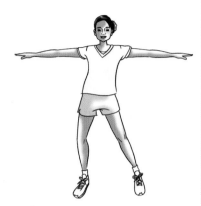

1 Step one leg out to the side, then bring the other to meet it. Now go back to the centre, and step the other way. Count out the steps – 'one, two, one two' – as you do it.

2 Now take two steps to the side, before coming back to the centre and going the other way. Stretch your arms out to the sides as you do it. Go a little faster, then slow down again.

Punch the piñata

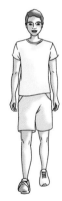
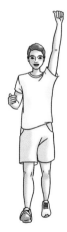

1 Stand with your feet about hip-distance apart. Step out first one foot then the other, so that each heel gently hits the floor, with your toes curling up towards the ceiling. Maintain a steady rhythm.

2 Once you have the heel digs going, bend the arms. Punch upwards with the opposite arm as you step – imagine you are whacking an invisible piñata. Keep going with alternate heel digs and punches for 1 minute.

MAKE IT FUN

• Put on some good dance music, and turn it up.
• Don't be afraid to be a sergeant major, albeit a happy one – do lots of 'hup, two, three, four' calls.
• Join in yourself – do all the actions. Your children can follow your lead, and they will enjoy working out with you.
• Don't do a single exercise for too long. Chop and change every minute or two to keep everyone interested.
• Try adapting the exercise names to something that tallies with young children's interests – if they are into witches and wizards, turn an aeroplane action into a swooping magical cloak.
• Motivate older children by repeating 'keep it going, you are halfway through', 'last few seconds – 10, 9, 8, 7, 6...' and the like.

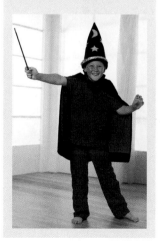

Hit your knee

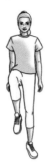 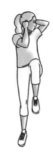

1 Standing on the spot, bend one leg and lift it into the air – high knees. Bend the opposite arm and bring the elbow to meet the knee. This gives you a good twist; great for flexibility.

2 Alternate the legs with every step. If you can meet the knee easily, try holding your ears, so your elbows are higher – this gets you lifting the knee even higher.

Kick your butt

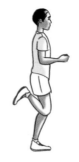 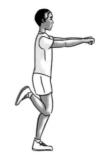

1 Stand with your feet shoulder-width apart. Move from one foot to the other, kicking the opposite leg up behind you as if you are trying to kick your own butt. Do this for 30 seconds.

2 Now add in some arm movements. As you move, stretch your arms out in front of you and then pull them towards you as you do the kick up to your butt.

Run on the spot

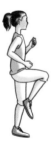 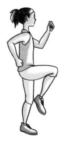

1 Increase the tempo by running on the spot for a full minute or two. Keep your children going by pretending you are running away from something – for example, you could say that some silly monsters are chasing you.

2 Pump your arms as you run, to turn this into a whole-body exercise. Describe various points on a known route – 'come on, we are at the newsagents'; 'now we are going up the hill to school' etc.

Bend to the side

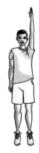 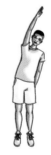

1 Stand with your feet shoulder-width apart. Stretch your arm high above your head and then bend to the side, like a tree in the wind.

2 Come back up to the middle and drop the raised arm, then lift the opposite arm and bend to the other side. Alternate between the two sides, working with a slow, gentle movement, for a minute or two.

Aeroplane

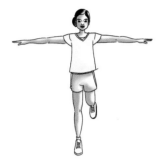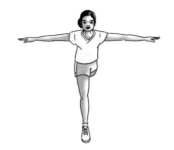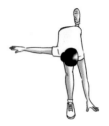

1 Stand on one leg, and balance for 10 seconds. Stretch your arms out to the sides, and then slowly bend forwards, keeping your balance. Stop briefly if you wobble, then carry on.

2 Keep your arms out for balance and let your bent leg come up behind you. Go as low as you can – like a swooping aeroplane. Focus on a spot on the ground to help you balance.

3 Now slowly come back up again. If you go very low, you may need to put a hand on the ground to steady yourself. Do this exercise three times, then repeat with the other leg.

Shoulder stretch

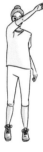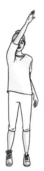

1 Stand with your feet at least hip-distance apart. Shift your weight to one side and reach one arm across your body as if you are reaching an apple on a branch that is high up and just out of reach. Repeat the action on the opposite side, reaching the other way.

2 Move from one side to the other, and vary the height of the things you are reaching for – high, middle, low. Pretend you are picking peaches from a tree, blackberries from a bush and strawberries from the ground. Shout out different fruits to change the stretch.

Clocks and windmills

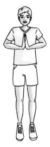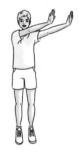

1 Put your hands together in front of you, fingers pointing up. Keeping your palms together, make circles with your arms – as if you are tracing round an imaginary clockface. Do this exercise for 15–30 seconds, then go the other way round.

2 Now take your hands apart, and have your palms facing away from you. Trace large circles in the air with your hands – as if they are the sails of a windmill. Do this for 15–20 seconds, then go back round the other way. Keep encouraging and praising your kids.

SPEED IT UP

This is a high-energy workout that introduces some slightly more complex exercises. Don't worry if your kids don't do them exactly as shown – so long as they aren't doing anything dangerous, the key thing is to keep them moving.

If you aren't using the exercise planners, do some warm-up exercises or running on the spot for a few minutes before trying these moves. Warming up raises the heart and respiratory rate and helps increase blood flow to the muscles, preparing them for more demanding routines.

It's not necessary to stretch before you work out – in fact, stretching out cold muscles makes them more susceptible to injury. The best way to warm up is to practise similar activities to the one you are about to do, but more slowly. Ideally, a warm-up will last 5 minutes or so.

Star jumps (jumping jacks)

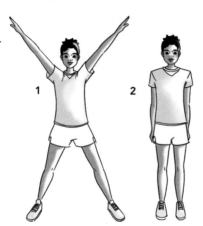

1 Stand with your feet together, arms by your side. Jump your feet out wide and stretch your arms out and up, so that your body forms a star shape.

2 Jump your feet back together and your arms by your sides. Keep going for 2 minutes – use the traffic light game (see box) to keep your kids interested.

The leg pendulum

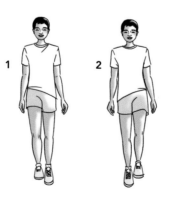

1 Stand on one leg, keeping the other leg straight. Slowly rock the hanging leg back and forth using large, controlled movements.

2 Gradually get quicker and quicker, using smaller and smaller movements. Swap to the other leg and repeat.

KEEPING THEM GOING
• Keep changing the speed at which you are working – ramp it up so that your children (and you) get slightly out of breath for a minute or two, then slow it down.
• Play traffic lights. Shout 'red light' to stop; 'green light' to go. This is a fantastic way to distract children from the fact that they are working quite hard. And the stop-start momentum makes everyone laugh.
• Get your children to suggest exercises that they do at school.

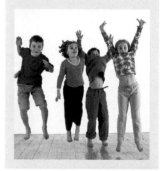

Swing out

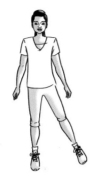 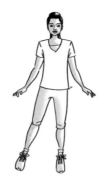

Pull-downs

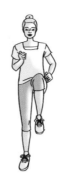 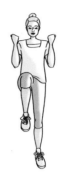

1 Similar to the leg pendulum, this exercise involves swinging first one leg then the other – this time to the side. Lift your leg out to the side (keeping your foot facing forwards and the leg straight), then bring it back to the centre before repeating with the other leg.

2 Start by doing this slowly in a controlled manner, but then go faster and faster, so that you are hopping from one leg to the other. Alternate between moving slowly and quickly – or play the traffic light game – in order to keep it going for 2 minutes.

1 It's time to speed things up again with a high-knees march. Start off with a brisk march, bringing the knees higher and higher with each step.

2 Now raise your arms above your head. As your knee comes up, pull the arms down to meet it. Do this for a full minute – it's another good one to do with the traffic light game as you end up in some hard-to-balance positions, which adds to the fun.

Walk like a creepy-crawly

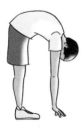 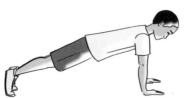 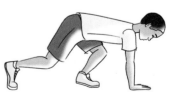

1 Stand with your feet hip–width apart. Bend over by dropping your head, neck, upper back and then lower back, and put your hands on the floor. Bend your knees if you need to.

2 Walk your hands forwards, leaving your feet where they are, until your heels come off the floor and your back is straight, as if you were about to do some press–ups.

3 Now slowly walk your feet to meet your hands – walk like a centipede – until you are in a bending position again. Repeat this action four or five times, travelling across the room.

Giant's steps

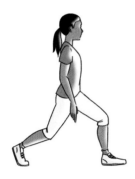 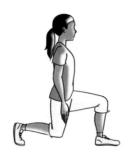 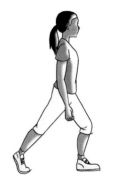

1 From standing, take a giant step forwards. Keep both feet pointing forwards – this is important as it helps to protect the knees (tell younger children that giants always keep their toes pointing in the same direction).

2 Bend the back knee towards the floor. Keep your hands by your sides and your back straight – giants have good posture – and make sure that your front knee doesn't move past your toes (this is important).

3 Come up slowly, and repeat the exercise five times, then repeat the action using the other leg.

Toe kicks

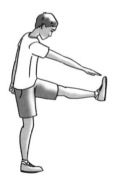 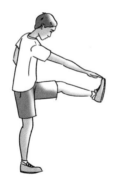

1 Stand with your feet hip-width apart, toes pointing forwards. Raise one leg in front of you, keeping it as straight as you can. Touch your toes with your opposite hand.

2 Alternate between exercising one side and then the other. If you find it hard to reach your toes with a straight leg, bend the knee of the raised leg a little.

Seal walking

1 This exercise is fantastic for building upper-body strength and maintaining flexibility in the spine. Get down on your hands and knees, then inch your hands forwards until your legs are stretched behind you and your back is upright – the Upward dog/ cobra position.

2 Use your hands to propel yourself forwards and move around the room, letting your legs drag along the floor behind you. Make seal barks as you move to encourage your kids to keep going. You will need quite a bit of space for this exercise, especially if several people are doing it.

Crab walking

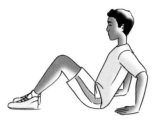

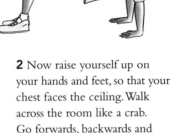

1 Sit down with your feet flat on the floor and your knees bent. Place your hands behind you, with your palms flat on the floor and your fingers pointing towards your feet. Your elbows will be slightly bent and you'll be leaning backwards.

2 Now raise yourself up on your hands and feet, so that your chest faces the ceiling. Walk across the room like a crab. Go forwards, backwards and sideways. Try designating a child to be the leader, and then follow them around.

Frog jumps

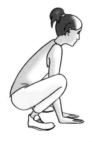

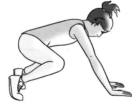

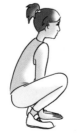

1 Getting down low is a fantastic way to keep the body flexible, and is a great strength-builder, too. Squat down, turning your toes outwards, and put your hands on the floor in front of you.

2 Now place your hands on the floor a little way in front of you, leaning forwards and coming up on to your toes. Jump your feet forwards around your hands – like a frog.

3 Move across the room in this way for a couple of minutes, making little hops and perhaps saying 'Gribbidd!' as you do so. This move is surprisingly energetic (as well as fun), and requires balance and coordination.

MOVING ON
• If you or your children find the exercises become very easy as you get fitter and stronger, you could increase the amount of time you do each one for, or up the number of repetitions; add some extra exercises to the routine; or even simply repeat the workout so you perform it twice in a row.
• Some of these exercises are the basis of dance routines, so once your children are confident doing them you could have a go at setting them to some up-tempo music. Or, even better, why not see if there is a dance class suitable for your child's age and encourage them to go along with some friends. If working out is seen as being a fun activity, children are generally much more inclined to stick with it.

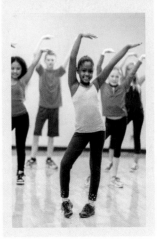

FASTER, FITTER, STRONGER

These are more intense than the previous exercises but should still be manageable for children as well as teenagers. Remind them to explore the exercises gently – there should be no forcing or holding a posture that hurts.

It's essential to warm up for 5–6 minutes before you do these exercises – use the previous routines or the exercise planners to prime yourself. To keep your kids warmed up and having fun, alternate these strength exercises with a few star jumps (jumping jacks) or marching. Make sure they aren't straining at any point – kids tend to be more resilient than most adults but they can still be injured if they overdo it. Take a few minutes at the end to cool down – to help your heart and respiratory rates to return to normal, and your muscles to relax. It's a way to help children transition to normal activity, too.

Make sure everyone does the exercises at their own pace; take breaks when you need to, and have some water to hand.

Curl-ups

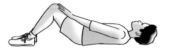 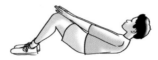

1 Lie flat on your back, with your knees bent and your feet hip-width apart and flat on the floor. Put your hands, palms down, on your thighs.

2 Breathe out as your curl up, lifting your shoulders a short distance from the floor, and then lower yourself back to the floor. Do this a few times.

Squats

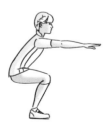 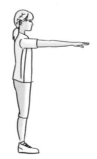

1 Stand with your feet hip-width apart. Bend your knees and lower your bottom, with a straight back, until your knees are bent. Stretch out your hands in front.

2 Come back up and repeat a few times. Your thighs should be parallel to the floor. Ensure that your knees go no further forwards than your toes.

EXERCISE OUTSIDE
You don't have to be at home or indoors in order to do some of these exercises – many can be done whenever you have a few minutes to spare, wherever you are. If the weather is good, you could go to the park to do a full workout routine, perhaps combining it with an active outdoor game, a brisk walk or a jog.

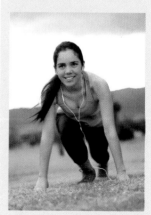

Kneeling push-ups

1 Push-ups are perfect for building upper-body strength. Go on your hands and knees, with your lower legs bent so that your feet are up in the air. Your hands should be positioned further apart than shoulder-width and your arms should be straight. Don't lock your elbows.

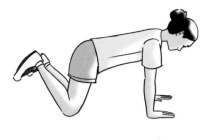

2 Pull in your tummy muscles, breathe in and bend your elbows to bring yourself as close to the ground as you can. Keep your back and neck straight and keep your tummy muscles tight. Hold this lower position for a count of three.

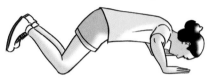

3 Breathe out as you straighten your arms and come back out of the push-up. Repeat eight times in total. If you find the exercise easy, you can make it harder by straightening your legs and coming up on your toes to the full press-up position (as shown in step 1 of Mountain climbing, below).

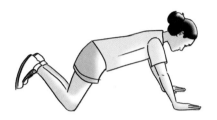

Mountain climbing

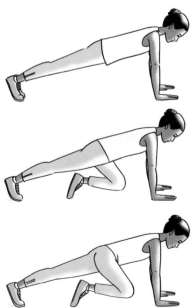

1 Lie face-down on the floor, with your hands further than shoulder-width apart and your legs stretched out behind you. Come up on your toes. Press your palms into the floor and come up into the full push-up position. Keep your back flat and pull in your tummy muscles.

2 Bring one knee forwards in a controlled manner as feels comfortable, then return it to the starting position and bring the other knee forwards. Try not to lift up your hips too much – it's a forwards rather than an upwards motion. Maintain a straight back and pull in your tummy muscles as you move your leg.

3 Keep going, getting quicker and quicker but still maintaining your posture and keeping your tummy muscles pulled in – this is a great exercise for upping the heart and respiratory rates. Keep going for a minute or so, then slow it down again.

Burpee

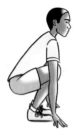 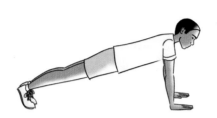 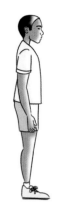

1 The name alone means most children will want to try this whole-body exercise. Stand up and then squat down, with your feet flat on the floor, bringing your hands to the floor in front of your feet.

2 Walk your feet back, until your legs and arms are straight and you are in the full push–up position (as shown). Hold the position for a count of three, maintaining a straight back.

3 Now walk your feet back to the starting position, and slowly stand up again. Repeat the exercise a few times, maintaining your form (eight times is great, but don't worry if you can't do that many yet).

Plank

1 Lie down on your front. Bend your arms so that you are resting on your 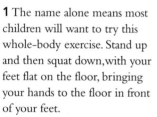 forearms. If you like, bring your palms together and interlace your fingers. Turn your toes under.

2 Push up on to your toes, keeping your back in a straight line with your head, 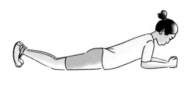 neck and legs. Hold for a few breaths, then release. Repeat three times, resting between each.

Triceps dips

1 Sit on the floor with your knees bent and your feet and hands flat 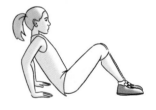 on the floor. Your hands should be slightly behind you, with your fingers pointing forwards.

2 Lift up your hips, bend your elbows and bring your upper body as close to 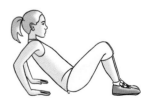 the floor as possible, then straighten your arms and bring yourself back up again. Repeat a few times.

Hang loose

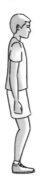 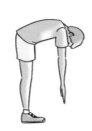

1 Start by standing with your feet about hip-width apart, feet facing forwards, and with your knees slightly bent. Relax your arms by your sides.

2 Fold from the waist and let your upper body and arms hang down. Breathe deeply, letting your body ease down with each exhale. Come up slowly, then repeat.

The stork

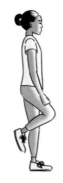 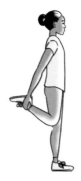

1 Stand on one leg, like a stork. Focus on a spot on the floor in front of you to help you keep your balance. If you really struggle, hold on to a chair.

2 Reach back, grasp your lifted foot, and bring it up towards your buttock (it doesn't have to touch). Take a few breaths, then release and do the other side.

Giant stretch

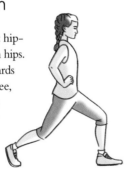

1 Stand with your feet hip-distance apart, hands on hips. Take a long step forwards and bend the front knee, making sure it doesn't poke forwards further than your toes. Bend the knee of the back leg slightly.

2 Straighten the back leg and then push the back foot flat on the floor. Keep your back straight and breathe. You should feel the stretch up the back of the back leg and in the thigh of the front one. Repeat on the other side.

Bent-leg stretch

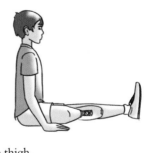

1 Sit on the floor with one leg straight out in front of you and the other bent with the knee facing outwards and the sole of your foot resting against the opposite thigh.

2 Reach towards the outstretched foot – breathe. Reach further into the stretch with each out-breath. Release, and repeat on the other side.

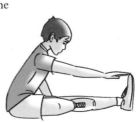

STRETCH IT OUT

Yoga exercises involve gentle movements and allow you to get in touch with your body. They also provide a fabulous way to help children wind down in the evening.

Remind your child to be gentle and not to force their body into a particular position, and don't try to adjust them – let them explore the moves in their own way. Encourage them to breathe fully throughout (see box). Show them the pose first, then talk them through the steps.

Downward dog

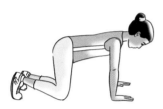 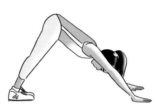 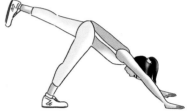

1 This fun pose gives the spine a great stretch. Get down on the floor, on your hands and knees, with your wrists under your shoulders and your knees under your hips. Spread your fingers wide. Turn your toes under.

2 Breathe out and lift your hips up to the ceiling at the same time as you straighten your legs. Let your head hang down, and take a few breaths – say 'woof woof!' as you do it.

3 Imagine you are wagging your tail as you shift your hips from side to side. Or try lifting one leg off the floor as if that is your tail, then do the other side. Breathe out, and come gently out of the pose.

Cat-to-cow pose

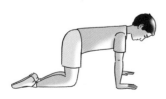 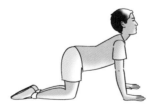 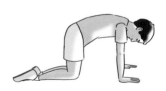

1 This is a good spine stretch. Go on your hands and knees, hands under shoulders and knees under hips – have your back flat like a table.

2 Breathe in, look up and lift your bottom upwards as you let your belly drop down, as if there are udders under there – say 'moo!' as you do it.

3 Breathe out, drop the head, tuck your tailbone under, and round your back – say 'miaow'. Go between the two poses, miaowing and mooing.

Upward dog/cobra pose

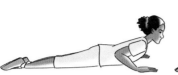

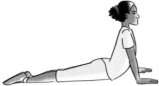

1 This is a gentle back bend that helps with posture and opens up the chest, promoting good breathing. Lie on your tummy on the floor with the tops of your feet on the floor. Place your hands palms-down underneath your shoulders. Your elbows will be bent and your chest should be slightly off the floor.

2 Breathing in, press your hands into the floor and lift up your upper body and head. Keep your elbows by your body and your legs straight so your kneecaps lift off the floor. Your back should be straight. Take a few breaths and then breathe in and return to the starting position on the floor. Repeat a few times.

AND BREATHE...
When you inhale, you should suck air all the way down into your tummy, which will move outwards. As you exhale, pull in your tummy muscles and empty your lungs of air before drawing the next breath. This is called 'belly breathing' and it aids relaxation and good oxygen flow around the body. Practise doing it when you exercise, coordinating breaths with the flow of the movements. Aim to breathe in as you exert yourself, and out as you relax.

Butterfly

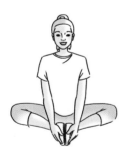

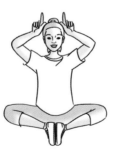

1 This is a calming pose, which helps to open up the hips. Sit on your bottom, and bring the soles of your feet together – knees out wide (your children may bring their knees closer to the floor than you can).

2 Slowly bring your knees up and down, as if you are fluttering your butterfly wings. Put your hands either side of your head, and point your forefingers upwards, waggling them as if they were your butterfly antennae.

Child's pose

1 This is a wonderfully soothing way to end a workout, since the pose gently stretches out the ankles, thighs and hips while allowing your body to relax. Kneel on the floor with your big toes together and your knees facing slightly outwards.

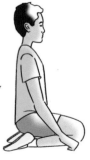

2 Breathing out, stretch down and rest your forehead on the floor, arms out in front of you or back by your feet (whatever feels right). Rest and relax, breathing naturally. Come out of the position slowly and take a few breaths.

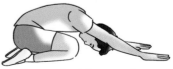

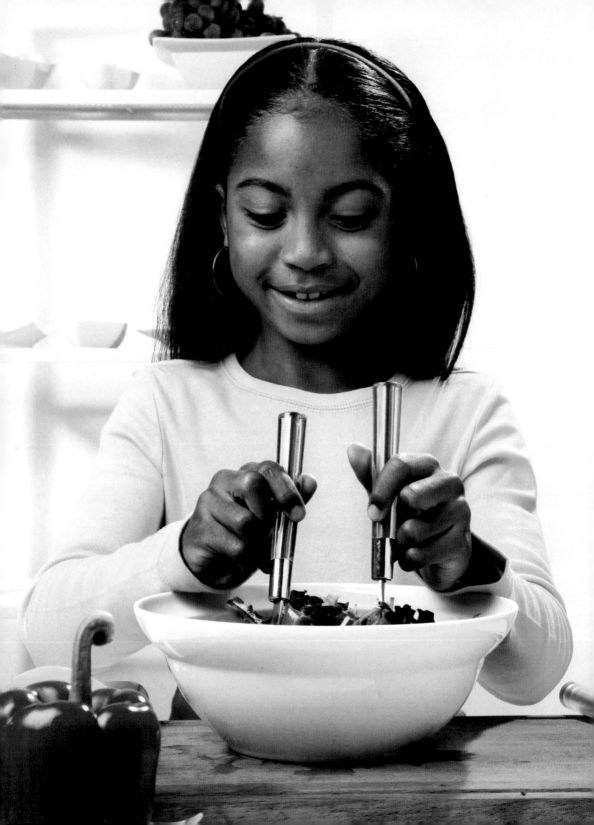

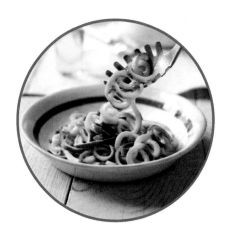

EATING WELL

As the old saying goes, we are what we eat, so it makes sense to feed ourselves the correct amount of nutritious, wholesome food. This section provides more than 100 delicious, nourishing dishes that cater to everyone's needs, whatever the time of day – from breakfasts, snacks and lunches to main meals, desserts and even the odd sweet treat.

BREAKFASTS AND DRINKS

Berry and quinoa porridge

Fibre-rich porridge keeps children going through the morning, and one study found that it helps with concentration at school. This one has added quinoa and vitamin-packed berries.

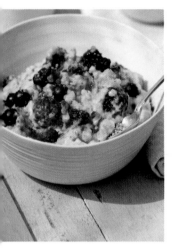

serves 4

300ml/½ pint/1¼ cups semi-skimmed (low-fat) milk or nut or soya milk
300ml/½ pint/1¼ cups water
115g/4oz/1 cup quinoa flakes
50g/2oz/½ cup rolled oats
115g/4oz/1 cup mixed berries, thawed
brown sugar, to serve (only if necessary)

1 Put the milk, water and quinoa flakes in a pan, bring to the boil and simmer for 5 minutes, until the flakes are softened.

2 Add the oats to the pan and simmer for a further 2 minutes, stirring often. Sprinkle the mixed berries over the top.

3 Cook the porridge for a further 2–3 minutes, until the berries are warmed through and just beginning to release their juices.

4 Serve the porridge immediately, sprinkled with some brown sugar and extra milk, if necessary.

Per portion Energy 166kcal/703kJ; Protein 7.6g; Carbohydrate 27.2g, of which sugars 3.6g; Fat 3.8g, of which saturates 0.3g; Cholesterol 0mg; Calcium 44mg; Fibre 1.9g; Sodium 48mg.

166 calories

Fresh and fruity muesli

Muesli is a brilliant breakfast booster that will keep you full until lunch. Use this recipe as a basic guide, but you can alter the balance of ingredients, or substitute others, if you like.

serves 2

1 pear
1 apple
1–2 plums
60ml/4 tbsp low-fat natural (plain) yogurt
60ml/2 tbsp grain flakes, such as barley, rye or rolled oats
15ml/1 tbsp ground nuts and/or seeds
15ml/1 tbsp raisins

1 Core and chop the pear and apple. Remove the stones (pits) from the plums and slice them.

2 Place the chopped fruit in a bowl and top with the yogurt then the grain flakes, nuts and raisins.

variations

• If you prefer the grain flakes to be soft rather than crunchy, try soaking them overnight in apple or orange juice to cover, or in a few tablespoons of water.
• Vary the fruit according to season. In the summer and autumn, use fresh soft fruit such as raspberries, strawberries, blackberries and blueberries. In the winter and spring, make the most of tropical fruits, such as pineapples, papayas, bananas, mangoes and kiwis. Be aware, however, that this will affect the nutritional data.

Per portion Energy 228kcal/963kJ; Protein 5.5g; Carbohydrate 41g, of which sugars 30g; Fat 12g, of which saturates 0.05g; Cholesterol 0.25mg; Calcium 87mg; Fibre 4.75g; Sodium 33mg.

228 calories

Granola and fruity yogurt toppings

Great for breakfast, this recipe also makes a lovely school snack: spoon some low-fat yogurt into a container then create a topping that can be stirred in just before the food is eaten. You can easily double the quantities and freeze the purée in an ice-cube tray so you can just thaw portions as you require them. The granola will keep for weeks in an airtight container.

each topping serves 4

for the raspberry and apple purée
1 eating apple, peeled and chopped
115g/4oz raspberries

for the apricot compote
3 ready-to-eat dried apricots, chopped
1 eating apple, peeled and chopped
1 nectarine, stoned (pitted) and chopped

for the granola
50g/2oz/½ cup rolled oats
50g/2oz/½ cup jumbo oats
25g/1oz/2 tbsp sunflower seeds
25g/1oz/2 tbsp sesame seeds
25g/1oz/2 tbsp roughly chopped hazelnuts
25g/1oz/¼ cup roughly chopped almonds
30ml/2 tbsp sunflower oil
30ml/2 tbsp clear honey
25g/1oz/2 tbsp raisins
25g/1oz/2 tbsp low-sugar dried cranberries

low-fat natural (plain) yogurt, to serve

1 To make the **raspberry and apple purée**, put the fruit in a pan with a little water. Cook over a low heat for 5 minutes, stirring until soft. Blend until smooth. Chill.

2 To make the **apricot compote**, put the fruit in a pan with a little water. Bring to the boil, reduce the heat and simmer for 10 minutes, until soft. Blend until smooth. Chill.

3 To make the **granola**, heat the oven to 140°C/ 275°F/Gas 1. Mix the oats, seeds and nuts in a bowl. Heat the oil and honey in a pan. Stir in the oat mixture. Spread out on baking sheets. Bake for 50 minutes, until crisp, tossing often. Transfer to a bowl. Stir in the raisins and cranberries. Leave to cool.

4 Swirl some of your chosen fruit topping into yogurt and top with granola.

Raspberry and apple purée: per portion Energy 68kcal/291kJ; Protein 4.8g; Carbohydrate 11.3g, of which sugars 11.3g; Fat 1g, of which saturates 0.5g; Cholesterol 1mg; Calcium 158mg; Fibre 2g; Sodium 65mg. **68** calories

Apricot compote: per portion Energy 139kcal/592kJ; Protein 6.4g; Carbohydrate 28.2g, of which sugars 28.2g; Fat 1.1g, of which saturates 0.4g; Cholesterol 1mg; Calcium 176mg; Fibre 3.7g; Sodium 69mg. **139** calories

Granola: per portion Energy 379kcal/1585kJ; Protein 9.9g; Carbohydrate 37.5g, of which sugars 17.85g; Fat 22.1g, of which saturates 2.25g; Cholesterol 0.5mg; Calcium 164mg; Fibre 3.7g; Sodium 49mg. **379** calories

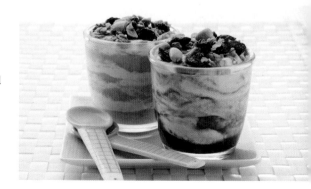

Apricot bran muffins

These moist, fruity muffins are a nutritious option for breakfast, especially if time is tight and you need to eat on the go. Apricots are packed with iron, fibre and vitamin A and their calcium content is further boosted by the yogurt and milk in the recipe. You can use nut milk and yogurt in place of dairy, if necessary.

makes 12

115g/4oz/1 cup dried apricots
225g/8oz/2 cups self-raising (self-rising) flour
50g/2oz/½ cup wheat or oat bran
2.5ml/½ tsp bicarbonate of soda (baking soda)
30ml/2 tbsp soft light brown sugar
30ml/2 tbsp unsalted butter, melted
150g/5oz/⅔ cup low-fat natural (plain) yogurt
200ml/7fl oz/scant 1 cup semi-skimmed (low-fat) milk

1 Grease the cups of a muffin tin or pan or line them with paper cases.

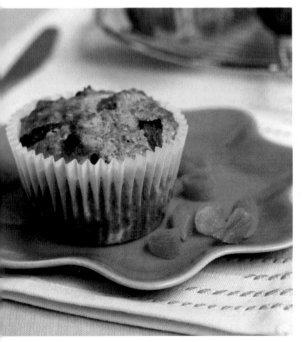

2 Soak the dried apricots in a small bowl of water for 15 minutes. Roughly chop the soaked apricots into small bitesize pieces.

3 Preheat the oven to 220°C/425°F/Gas 7.

4 In a large bowl, mix together the flour, bran, bicarbonate of soda, sugar and chopped apricots.

5 Add the melted butter, yogurt and milk to the bowl of dry ingredients. Mix lightly.

6 Two-thirds fill the prepared paper cases with batter. Bake for 15–20 minutes, until a skewer inserted into the centre of one comes out clean.

7 Leave the muffins to cool for 5 minutes, then turn out on to a wire rack to cool completely. Serve warm or store in an airtight container and eat within 2 days.

variation

• Replace the apricots with an equal quantity of other dried fruits, such as dates, raisins, sultanas (golden raisins) or cherries. It is important to soak whichever dried fruit you choose to use for about 15 minutes, otherwise the fruit would absorb liquid from the batter and affect its consistency, resulting in very dry and crumbly muffins that won't rise properly.

Per portion Energy 127kcal/539kJ; Protein 3.8g; Carbohydrate 22.7g, of which sugars 7.8g; Fat 3g, of which saturates 1.6g; Cholesterol 7mg; Calcium 119mg; Fibre 3.6g; Sodium 126mg.

127
calories

Apple fritters

These fruity little fritters are made with wholemeal flour for fibre and only a little honey for sweetness, making them a healthy breakfast treat.

makes 12

2 eating apples, peeled, cored and coarsely grated
140g/4¾oz/scant 1¼ cups strong white bread flour, plus extra for dusting
140g/4¾oz/scant 1¼ cups strong wholemeal (whole-wheat) bread flour
5ml/1 tsp baking powder
a pinch of salt
275ml/9fl oz/generous 1 cup lukewarm water
15ml/1 tbsp clear honey
1 egg
about 30ml/2 tbsp sunflower oil, for frying

1 Squeeze out any moisture from the grated apple using kitchen paper. Set aside.

2 Sift the flours together with the baking powder and salt into a large bowl. Add the water, honey, egg and grated apples and stir to combine.

3 Heat the oil in a large frying pan. Working in batches of three, drop about 30ml/2 tbsp of batter for each fritter into the hot oil, and cook for 30–60 seconds on each side, until golden brown all over.

4 Remove from the oil using a slotted spoon or fish slice, and drain on kitchen paper. Keep warm while you cook the remaining fritters. Serve the fritters warm.

Per portion Energy 75kcal/314kJ; Protein 1.7g; Carbohydrate 12.1g, of which sugars 3.1g; Fat 2.5g, of which saturates 0.4g; Cholesterol 16mg; Calcium 23mg; Fibre 0.9g; Sodium 46mg.

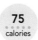
75 calories

Buttermilk pancakes

Home-made pancakes are lovely for a special-occasion breakfast, and are much healthier than pastries such as croissants, or a fry-up.

serves 6

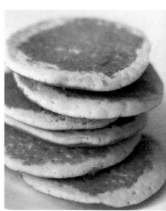

50g/2oz/½ cup plain (all-purpose) flour
50g/2oz/½ cup wholemeal (whole-wheat) flour
10ml/1 tsp baking powder
2 eggs
300ml/½ pint/1¼ cups buttermilk, or semi-skimmed milk and
5ml/1 tsp lemon juice
30ml/2 tbsp oil, for frying

1 Sift the flours and baking powder into a large bowl. Add the eggs and beat until smooth. Still beating, pour in enough buttermilk or milk mixed with lemon juice to make a thick, smooth batter.

2 Heat a frying pan, then add enough oil to just coat the base. Drop three or four tablespoonfuls of the mixture, spaced slightly apart, on to the pan.

3 Cook the pancakes over a medium heat for about 1 minute, or until the bottoms are golden brown. Flip the pancakes over and cook for a further 1 minute until both sides are cooked.

4 Cover the cooked pancakes with a clean dish towel while you cook the remaining pancake batter in the same way.

Per portion Energy 106kcal/446kJ; Protein 6.1g; Carbohydrate 14.9g, of which sugars 2.8g; Fat 2.8g, of which saturates 0.8g; Cholesterol 78mg; Calcium 105mg; Fibre 1.4g; Sodium 253mg.

106 calories

Eggtastic

These two classic egg recipes are worth perfecting as they can be eaten for breakfast, lunch or as a healthy snack. Cook the eggs through for younger children, if you prefer.

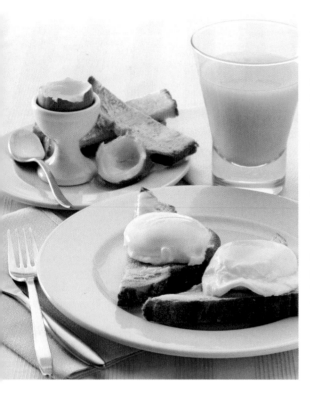

1 To make the **dippy egg with toast soldiers**, put the egg in a pan and pour in hot water to cover.

2 Bring to the boil and cook for 3 minutes for a very soft egg or 4 minutes for a soft yolk and firm white.

3 Remove the egg from the water with a slotted spoon and place it in an egg cup.

4 Meanwhile, make the soldiers. Toast the bread, spread it lightly with butter, then cut it into fingers. Serve with the boiled egg.

5 For the **poached eggs on toast**, three–quarters fill a frying pan with hot water. Heat gently, until it is just simmering, then add the lemon juice or vinegar. If you have egg poaching rings, add them to the pan.

6 Crack the eggs into the pan or rings. Cook for 2–3 minutes, until the eggs are white and just set.

7 Meanwhile, lightly toast the bread and spread it with a little butter. Remove the poached eggs from the pan with a slotted spoon, being careful not to break the yolks. Arrange the poached eggs on the toast and serve immediately.

each serves 1

dippy egg with toast soldiers (sticks)
1 egg
2 slices bread, preferably wholemeal (whole-wheat)
a little unsalted butter, for spreading

poached eggs on toast
2 eggs
5ml/1 tsp lemon juice or vinegar
2 slices bread, preferably wholemeal (whole-wheat)
a little unsalted butter, for spreading

Dippy egg with toast soldiers: per portion Energy 245kcal/1030kJ; Protein 11.7g; Carbohydrate 24.7g, of which sugars 1.3g; Fat 11.8g, of which saturates 4.7g; Cholesterol 242mg; Calcium 90mg; Fibre 1g; Sodium 374mg.

245 calories

Poached eggs on toast: per portion Energy 336kcal/1406kJ; Protein 19.2g; Carbohydrate 24.7g, of which sugars 1.3g; Fat 18.5g, of which saturates 6.6g; Cholesterol 473mg; Calcium 124mg; Fibre 1g; Sodium 458mg.

336 calories

Ham and tomato scramble

Scrambled egg isn't just for breakfast – it makes a delicious and easy lunch or snack. Only a small amount of ham is used, adding a protein boost but not much fat or salt.

serves 2

2 slices good-quality ham
1 tomato
¼ red (bell) pepper, seeded
2 eggs
15ml/1 tbsp semi-skimmed (low-fat) milk
15ml/1 tbsp unsalted butter
2 slices bread, preferably wholemeal (whole-wheat)

1 Finely chop the ham on a chopping board. Halve the tomato, scoop out and discard the seeds, then chop the flesh finely. Finely chop the pieces of pepper.

2 Put the eggs and milk in a bowl and whisk lightly with a fork.

3 Heat a small pat of the butter in a pan over a medium heat, until it is just foaming. Do not let it brown.

4 Add the egg mixture with the ham, tomato and pepper and cook gently, stirring all the time, over a low heat for about 3 minutes. Remove from the heat. Take care not to overcook the eggs or they will become rubbery.

5 Lightly toast the bread, then spread it with the remaining butter. Cut the toast into shapes with small novelty-shaped cookie cutters, if you like (see cook's tips).

6 Arrange the toast on serving plates, spoon over the ham and tomato scramble and serve immediately. You can easily double or even treble the quantities to feed more people.

cook's tips

• This is a good breakfast treat for themed days, such as Halloween or Valentine's Day, if you use appropriate-shaped cutters for the toast. If you don't have special cutters, simply cut the toast into shapes with a knife.
• Add any of your favourite vegetables, such as corn or peas, to the scramble.

Per portion Energy 350kcal/1456kJ; Protein 14.1g; Carbohydrate 17.1g, of which sugars 4.4g; Fat 25.7g, of which saturates 14.3g; Cholesterol 257mg; Calcium 78mg; Fibre 1.3g; Sodium 689mg.

350 calories

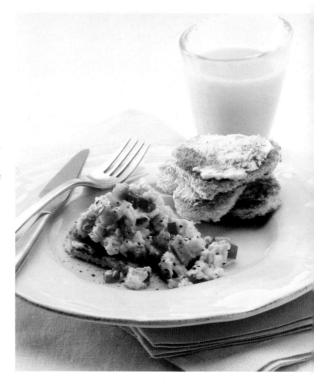

Mango and lime lassi

This tangy, fruity blend of ripe mango, cooling yogurt and sharp, fresh lime juice makes a satisfying drink.

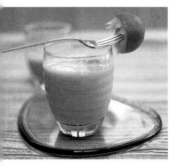

serves 3

1 mango
finely grated rind and
    juice of 1 lime
clear honey, to taste
100ml/3½fl oz/scant
    ½ cup low-fat natural
    (plain) yogurt
chilled water, to dilute

1 Peel the mango and cut the flesh from the stone (pit). Put the flesh into a food processor or blender and add the lime rind and juice.

2 Add honey to taste, and the yogurt. Whizz the mixture until it is completely smooth, scraping down the sides once or twice.

3 Stir a little chilled water into the lassi mixture to thin it down to the required consistency for drinking. Serve immediately.

cook's tip

• Yogurt adds calcium to this lassi, and the protein will help make it more sustaining.

variation

• You can use drained canned mango, peaches or apricots in natural juice in place of the fresh fruit.

Per portion Energy 63kcal/268kJ; Protein 2g; Carbohydrate 13.6g, of which sugars 13.5g; Fat 0.4g, of which saturates 0.3g; Cholesterol 0mg; Calcium 60mg; Fibre 1.7g; Sodium 23mg.

63 calories

Raspberry smoothie

A vibrant blend of raspberries and orange mixed with yogurt makes a great after-school pick-you-up.

serves 3

250g/9oz/1⅓ cups raspberries
200ml/7fl oz/scant 1 cup low-fat natural
    (plain) yogurt
300ml/½ pint/1¼ cups unsweetened freshly
    squeezed orange juice

1 Chill the raspberries, yogurt and orange juice in the refrigerator for about 1 hour before you make the drink.

2 Place the raspberries and yogurt in a blender or food processor. Blend together thoroughly until smooth, scraping the mixture down with a spatula, if necessary.

3 Alternatively, if you don't have a blender or food processor, or you'd prefer not to have the little raspberry seeds in your drink, press the raspberries through a sieve or strainer, collecting the purée in a bowl positioned below. Add the yogurt to the raspberry purée in the bowl and stir to combine thoroughly.

4 Add the orange juice and process for another 30 seconds. Or, if you have used the sieve/strainer method for the raspberries, stir in the orange juice until combined.

5 Pour the smoothie into glasses and serve immediately with straws, if you like.

Per portion Energy 94kcal/403kJ; Protein 4.9g; Carbohydrate 17.6g, of which sugars 17.6g; Fat 1g, of which saturates 0.5g; Cholesterol 1mg; Calcium 139mg; Fibre 2.9g; Sodium 55mg.

94 calories

Creamy banana boost

A luscious blend of banana, pineapple, dates, lemon juice and milk, this delicious concoction will keep you going for hours.

serves 3

½ pineapple
4 Medjool dates, stoned (pitted)
1 small ripe banana
juice of 1 lemon
300ml/½ pint/1¼ cups very cold skimmed milk

1 Using a small, sharp knife, cut away the skin and core from the pineapple. Roughly chop the flesh and put it in a blender or food processor, then add the stoned dates.

2 Peel and chop the banana and add it to the rest of the fruit together with the lemon juice.

3 Blend thoroughly until smooth, stopping to scrape the mixture down from the side of the bowl with a rubber spatula, if necessary.

4 Add the milk to the blender or food processor and process briefly until well combined. Pour the smoothie into tall glasses and serve immediately.

variations

• You can use soya or any kind of nut or seed milk instead of dairy milk if you prefer. Nut and seed milks will lend the blend a subtle flavour as well as adding nutrients.
• Dates are a great way to add natural sweetness, but you could also use ready-to-eat dried apricots.

Per portion Energy 170kcal/725kJ; Protein 4.4g; Carbohydrate 39.4g, of which sugars 38.8g; Fat 0.5g, of which saturates 0.1g; Cholesterol 2mg; Calcium 138mg; Fibre 3.8g; Sodium 45mg.

170 calories

Banana and mango thickie

Vitamin C-rich orange juice and sweet, scented mango in this drink will get your tastebuds tingling first thing.

serves 3

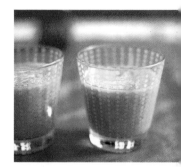

1 ripe mango
1 large banana
1 large juicy
   orange
15ml/1 tbsp sesame
   seeds (optional)
chilled water, to dilute
   (optional)

1 Using a small, sharp knife, skin the mango, then slice the flesh off the stone (pit).

2 Peel the banana and break it into lengths, then place it in a blender or food processor with the mango flesh.

3 Squeeze the juice from the orange and add it to the blender or food processor along with the sesame seeds, if using.

4 Whizz until the mixture is smooth, then pour into glasses and serve. You can dilute the drink to serve more people by adding water, if you like.

cook's tip

• Sesame seeds not only taste delicious, but they also provide a good source of vitamin E, as well as some calcium. For extra fibre value, add 25ml/ 1½ tbsp medium oatmeal to the smoothie.

Per portion 148Kcal/625kJ; Protein 3.1g; Carbohydrate 25g, of which sugars 23.9g; Fat 4.7g, of which saturates 0.8g; Cholesterol 0mg; Calcium 90mg; Fibre 4g; Sodium 7mg.

148 calories

LUNCHES

Hummus

Hummus is perfect for a packed lunch or picnic, served with some pitta bread, crusty bread or vegetable sticks.

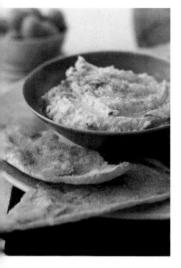

400g/14oz can
    chickpeas, drained
1 garlic clove, peeled
30ml/2 tbsp tahini or
    sugar-free no-salt
    smooth peanut butter
60ml/4 tbsp olive oil
juice of 1 lemon
2.5ml/½ tsp cayenne
    pepper (optional), plus
    extra for sprinkling
toasted pitta or crusty
    bread or vegetable
    sticks, to serve

1 Rinse the chickpeas in a colander or strainer, then tip them into a blender or food processor with the garlic. Blend until the mixture is almost a smooth paste.

2 Add the tahini or peanut butter and blend until fairly smooth. With the motor running, pour in the oil and lemon juice.

3 Stir in the cayenne pepper, if you are using it. If the mixture is too thick, stir in a little water.

4 Transfer the hummus to a serving bowl or a lidded plastic container for a packed lunch. Sprinkle over some cayenne pepper, if liked.

Per portion Energy 151kcal/629kJ; Protein 4.6g; Carbohydrate 8.2g, of which sugars 0.2g; Fat 11.3g, of which saturates 1.5g; Cholesterol 0mg; Calcium 22mg; Fibre 2.8g; Sodium 110mg.

151
calories

Carrot dip

This delicious dip combines the sweet taste of carrots and oranges with the light spiciness of a mild curry paste.

serves 4–6

1 onion, peeled
3 carrots
grated rind and juice of 2 oranges
15ml/1 tbsp mild curry paste
150ml/¼ pint/⅔ cup low-fat natural (plain) yogurt
a handful of fresh basil leaves
15–30ml/1–2 tbsp fresh lemon juice, to taste
ground black pepper, to taste
celery and cucumber sticks, to serve

1 Finely chop the onion. Peel and grate the carrots, then place the onion, carrots, orange rind and juice, and curry paste in a small pan. Bring to the boil, cover and simmer gently for 10 minutes, until the vegetables are tender.

2 Transfer the mixture to a blender or food processor and process until it is smooth. Leave it to cool completely.

3 Stir in the yogurt, then tear the basil leaves into small pieces and stir them into the carrot mixture so that everything is combined. Add the lemon juice and season with pepper.

4 Transfer the dip to a serving bowl or a lidded plastic container for a packed lunch. Chill in the refrigerator until shortly before serving, then allow it to come to room temperature. Serve with celery and cucumber sticks.

Per portion Energy 51kcal/213kJ; Protein 2g; Carbohydrate 9g, of which sugars 8.1g; Fat 1g, of which saturates 0.2g; Cholesterol 0mg; Calcium 63mg; Fibre 1.9g; Sodium 67mg.

51
calories

Artichoke and cumin dip

High-fibre artichokes can be blitzed to make a low-calorie, low-fat creamy dip that children will enjoy eating.

serves 4

400g/14oz can artichoke hearts
1 garlic clove, peeled
2.5ml/½ tsp ground cumin
olive oil
ground black pepper, to taste
selection of raw vegetable crudités, to serve

1 Drain the artichoke hearts, reserving the oil for salad dressings.

2 Put the artichoke hearts in a food processor with the garlic, ground cumin and a drizzle of olive oil. Process to a smooth purée and season with black pepper to taste.

3 Transfer the dip to a small serving bowl or a lidded plastic container for a packed lunch. Serve with a selection of raw vegetable crudités, for dipping.

cook's tips

• Using spices such as ground cumin in this dip means that you do not need to add salt. Lemon juice and fresh herbs also add flavour, so try replacing salt with these in other dishes too and see how they taste.
• For extra flavour, add a handful of fresh basil leaves to the artichokes before blending them in the food processor.

Per portion Energy 40kcal/165kJ; Protein 2.3g; Carbohydrate 2.2g, of which sugars 1g; Fat 2.9g, of which saturates 0.5g; Cholesterol 0mg; Calcium 33mg; Fibre 0.1g; Sodium 11mg.

40 calories

Peanut dip

This coconutty satay dip can be served with strips of raw or roasted vegetables, or strips of cooked chicken.

serves 4

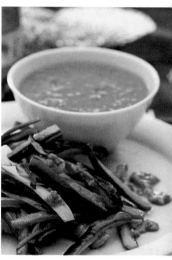

40g/1½oz creamed
  coconut, chopped
60ml/4 tbsp sugar-free
  no-salt crunchy
  peanut butter
15ml/1 tbsp soy sauce
1.5ml/¼ tsp dried chilli
  flakes (optional)
1 garlic clove, crushed
5ml/1 tsp finely grated
  lemon rind
**strips of raw or roasted
  vegetables, to serve**

1 Put the chopped creamed coconut in a heatproof bowl and pour over 300ml/½ pint/1¼ cups boiling water. Stir until dissolved.

2 Add the peanut butter, soy sauce, dried chilli flakes (if using), garlic and finely grated lemon rind and stir to combine everything to a smooth dip. Leave the dip to cool and thicken slightly at room temperature.

3 Transfer the peanut dip to a serving bowl or a lidded plastic container for a packed lunch. Serve it with a selection of raw vegetable crudités or some strips of roasted vegetables or chicken, for dipping.

Per portion Energy 177kcal/737kJ; Protein 4.6g; Carbohydrate 4.7g, of which sugars 1g; Fat 16.5g, of which saturates 7g; Cholesterol 0mg; Calcium 3mg; Fibre 2.9g; Sodium 270mg.

177 calories

Cheese and potato bread twists

If you like cheese sandwiches, you'll love these cheesy twists. They are delicious served warm at home or cold in a packed lunch, and children will enjoy helping to knead the dough. If you are pushed for time you could also try using a low-salt bread mix and adding some leftover mashed potato. They also freeze well.

makes 8
. . . .

225g/8oz potatoes, peeled, diced and boiled
115g/4oz/1 cup strong white bread flour
115g/4oz/1 cup strong wholemeal (whole-wheat)
   bread flour
5ml/1 tsp easy-blend (rapid-rise) dried yeast
a pinch of salt
150ml/¼ pint/⅔ cup lukewarm water,
175g/6oz/1½ cups finely grated low-fat
   red Leicester or Cheddar cheese

1 Mash the potatoes until smooth and set aside. Sift the flours into a bowl and add the yeast and a pinch of salt.

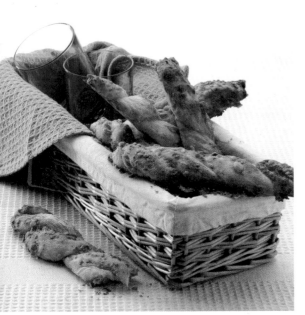

2 Stir in the potatoes and rub with your fingers until the mixture resembles breadcrumbs.

3 Make a well in the centre and pour in the lukewarm water. Bring the mixture together with your hands.

4 Knead for 5 minutes on a floured surface. Return to the bowl, cover with a damp cloth and leave to rise in a warm place for 1 hour, until doubled in size.

5 Turn out on to the work surface and re-knead the dough for a few seconds. Divide it into 8 equal-size pieces and shape into balls.

6 Scatter the cheese over a clean surface, such as a large chopping board or tray. Roll each ball of dough in the cheese.

7 Roll each ball on a dry surface to form a long sausage shape. Fold the two ends together and twist the bread. Lay these on a baking sheet lined with baking parchment.

8 Cover the twists with a damp cloth and leave to rise in a warm place for 30 minutes.

9 Preheat the oven to 220°C/425°F/Gas 7. Bake the twists for 10–15 minutes, until risen and golden. Serve warm or cold.

. . . .
Per portion Energy 197kcal/829kJ; Protein 8.2g; Carbohydrate 26.9g, of which sugars 0.8g; Fat 7g, of which saturates 4.2g; Cholesterol 27mg; Calcium 181mg; Fibre 1.6g; Sodium 140mg.

197
calories

Cheese straws

A little cheese goes a long way in these crunchy, flavoursome snacks. Serve with healthy dips or perhaps some vegetable-packed soup.

makes 10

40g/1½oz/⅓ cup plain (all-purpose) flour
40g/1½oz/⅓ cup plain wholemeal (all-purpose whole-wheat) flour
ground black pepper, to taste
40g/1½oz/3 tbsp unsalted butter, diced
40g/1½oz low-fat mature (sharp) hard cheese, such as Cheddar, finely grated
1 egg
5ml/1 tsp ready-made mustard

1 Preheat the oven to 180°C/350°F/Gas 4. Line a baking sheet with baking parchment.

2 Sift the flours and pepper into a large bowl. Rub the butter into the flour until the mixture resembles fine crumbs. Stir in the cheese.

3 Lightly beat the egg with the mustard. Add half the egg to the flour, stirring in just enough so that the mixture can be gathered into a smooth ball of dough. Roll the dough out to make a square measuring about 15cm/6in. Cut into 10 lengths.

4 Place on the baking sheet lined with baking parchment and brush with the remaining egg. Bake for about 12 minutes, until golden brown.

5 Transfer to a wire rack and serve warm, or leave to cool and pack up with some dips for lunch.

Per portion Energy 77kcal/319kJ; Protein 3g; Carbohydrate 5.7g, of which sugars 0.2g; Fat 4.8g, of which saturates 2.7g; Cholesterol 33mg; Calcium 45mg; Fibre 0.7g; Sodium 74mg.

77 calories

Oatcakes

These high-fibre savoury home-made oatcakes are an ideal quick snack. Simply spread with hummus, cottage cheese or a dip, and serve with grapes.

makes 18

75g/3oz/⅔ cup plain wholemeal (all-purpose whole-wheat) flour
2.5ml/½ tsp salt
1.5ml/¼ tsp baking powder
115g/4oz/1 cup fine pinhead oatmeal
75g/3oz/6 tbsp white vegetable fat (shortening)

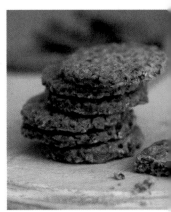

1 Preheat the oven to 200°C/400°F/Gas 6 and grease a baking sheet.

2 Sift the flour, salt and baking powder into a mixing bowl. Add the oatmeal and mix well. Rub in the fat to make a crumbly mixture. Gradually add water to the dry ingredients, mixing in just enough to make a stiff dough.

3 Turn out the dough on to a worktop sprinkled with fine oatmeal, and knead until smooth. Roll out to about 3mm/⅛in thick and cut into rounds, squares or triangles. Place on the baking sheets.

4 Bake for 15 minutes, until crisp. Cool the oatcakes on a wire rack. Store in an airtight container lined with a piece of baking parchment.

Per portion Energy 70kcal/291kJ; Protein 1.3g; Carbohydrate 7.3g, of which sugars 0.1g; Fat 4.1g, of which saturates 1.7g; Cholesterol 1mg; Calcium 6mg; Fibre 1.1g; Sodium 91mg.

70 calories

Cheesy quesadilla

Kids love these simple toasted flatbreads, and you can use any number of fillings.

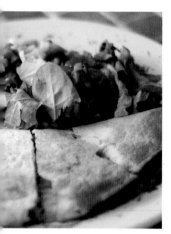

serves 1

30ml/2 tbsp grated or finely chopped low-fat mozzarella
30ml/2 tbsp grated low-fat hard cheese, such as Cheddar
1 spring onion (scallion), diced
1 tomato, finely diced
1 soft wholemeal (whole-wheat) tortilla
mixed salad, to serve

1 Mix together all the ingredients apart from the tortilla and salad. Heat a large frying pan over a medium heat, then lay the tortilla flat in it.

2 Spoon the filling on one half of the tortilla, leaving a small rim clear. Fold over the tortilla to form a semicircle and press down with a spatula.

3 Cook for 3–4 minutes, until golden brown underneath, then flip over and cook for a further 3–4 minutes to brown the other side. Cut into wedges and serve immediately with mixed salad.

variations

• Try filling with Tomato and lentil dhal (see page 124), or Giant baked beans (see page 125), adding a little grated cheese so it sticks together.

Per portion Energy 325kcal/1368kJ; Protein 19.7g; Carbohydrate 39.9g, of which sugars 3.1g; Fat 10.7g, of which saturates 6.6g; Cholesterol 27mg; Calcium 419mg; Fibre 3.1g; Sodium 486mg.

325 calories

Chicken pitta pockets

These scrummy pittas make a perfect substantial snack or weekend lunch.

serves 6

1 small cucumber
2 spring onions (scallions)
3 tomatoes
30ml/2 tbsp olive oil
30ml/2 tbsp finely chopped parsley
30ml/2 tbsp finely chopped mint
ground black pepper, to taste
45–60ml/3–4 tbsp tahini
juice of 1 lemon
2 garlic cloves, peeled and crushed
6 wholemeal (whole-wheat) pitta breads
2 roasted chicken breast fillets, flesh removed from the bone and cut into strips

1 Chop the cucumber, spring onions and tomatoes into small chunks and put them in a bowl. Stir in the oil, parsley and mint and season to taste with black pepper. Set aside.

2 In a second bowl, mix the tahini with the lemon juice, then thin down the mixture by stirring in a little water, until it has the consistency of thick double (heavy) cream. Beat in the crushed garlic with a fork.

3 Preheat the grill (broiler) to hot. Lightly toast the pittas, not too close to the heat, until they puff up.

4 Open the pittas and stuff them with the chicken and salad. Drizzle tahini sauce into each one and serve with any extra salad.

Per portion Energy 402kcal/1697kJ; Protein 23.3g; Carbohydrate 54.6g, of which sugars 5g; Fat 11.6g, of which saturates 1.8g; Cholesterol 35mg; Calcium 222mg; Fibre 4.5g; Sodium 456mg.

402 calories

Eggstra special sandwich selection

A delicious sandwich makes a convenient packed lunch, picnic or after-school snack. Egg is always a favourite, so why not learn the basics with these two great fillings.

serves 4

12 slices white or wholemeal (whole-wheat) bread
50g/2oz/¼ cup low-fat spread, at room temperature

for the egg and cress filling
2 eggs
30ml/2 tbsp low-fat mayonnaise
½ carton cress
ground black pepper, to taste

for the egg and tuna filling
2 eggs
75g/3oz drained canned tuna in spring water
5ml/1 tsp paprika
a squeeze of lemon juice
ground black pepper, to taste
25g/1oz piece cucumber, peeled and
   thinly sliced

1 To make the **egg and cress filling**, fill a pan with water and bring it to the boil. Carefully lower in the eggs, bring the water back to the boil and boil the eggs for 8 minutes.

2 Place the pan under running water for a few minutes, until the eggs are cool. Remove from the water and leave until completely cold, then tap on a hard surface and peel away the shells.

3 Finely chop the eggs, then place them in a bowl and add the mayonnaise, cress and ground black pepper to taste. Mix well.

4 To make the **egg and tuna filling**, first cook the eggs in the same way as for the egg and cress filling.

5 Put the tuna in a bowl and flake it with a fork. Mix in the eggs, paprika, lemon juice and pepper.

6 To make the sandwiches, you can start by removing the bread crusts, if you like. Then cover each slice of bread with a thin layer of spread.

7 Take half the slices: spread the egg and cress filling on half of these; and the egg and tuna filling on the other half, topping with cucumber. Lay the remaining bread slices on top. Cut into triangles and serve, or wrap in clear film or plastic wrap and chill.

Egg and cress: per portion Energy 179kcal/753kJ; Protein 7.1g; Carbohydrate 20.6g, of which sugars 1.4g; Fat 8.2g, of which saturates 3g; Cholesterol 98mg; Calcium 60mg; Fibre 0.9g; Sodium 354mg.

179 calories

Egg and tuna: per portion Energy 180kcal/759kJ; Protein 11.6g; Carbohydrate 20.5g, of which sugars 1.2g; Fat 6.4g, of which saturates 2.7g; Cholesterol 106mg; Calcium 64mg; Fibre 0.9g; Sodium 344mg.

180 calories

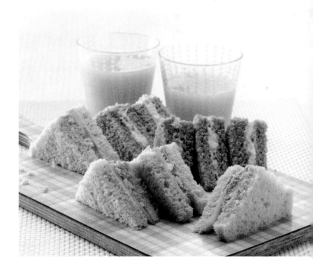

Cheese and ham tarts

These tasty little tarts are protein-rich, so they will keep kids full for a long time. They make a great alternative to sandwiches once in a while and freeze well.

makes 12

for the pastry
50g/2oz/½ cup plain (all-purpose) flour
50g/2oz/½ cup plain wholemeal (all-purpose whole-wheat) flour
50g/2oz/4 tbsp hard baking margarine, cubed

for the filling
50g/2oz/½ cup low-fat hard cheese, grated
2 thin slices good-quality ham, chopped
75g/3oz/½ cup frozen or drained canned corn
1 egg
120ml/4fl oz/½ cup semi-skimmed (low-fat) milk
a pinch of paprika
carrot and cucumber sticks, to serve

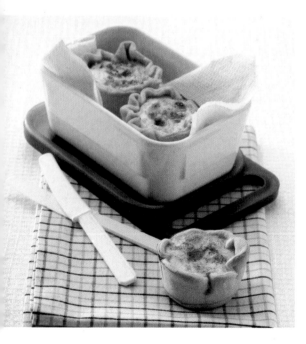

1 To make the pastry, place the flours in a bowl and add the margarine. Using your fingertips, rub the margarine into the flour until the mixture resembles breadcrumbs. Gradually add 20ml/4 tsp cold water and mix to a smooth dough with a palette or table knife.

2 Form the dough into a ball, then wrap it in clear film or plastic wrap and chill for 20 minutes.

3 Preheat the oven to 200°C/400°F/Gas 6. Lightly knead the pastry on to a floured surface. Using a rolling pin, roll it out thinly.

4 Stamp out 12 circles with a cutter, re-rolling the pastry trimmings as necessary. Press into the holes of a bun tin or pan. Chill for 30 minutes.

5 To make the filling, combine the cheese, ham and corn. Divide the mixture among the tarts. Beat together the egg and milk, pour into the tarts and sprinkle the tops with paprika.

6 Cook for 12–15 minutes, until the tarts are risen and browned. Cool slightly before loosening and sliding out with a palette knife. Serve warm or cold with carrot and cucumber sticks, or wrap in clear film or plastic wrap to transport.

cook's tip

• Home-made pastry is much healthier than store-bought types, and is easy to make.

Per portion Energy 93kcal/389kJ; Protein 4.3g; Carbohydrate 7.5g, of which sugars 0.8g; Fat 5.3g, of which saturates 2.5g; Cholesterol 25mg; Calcium 57mg; Fibre 0.8g; Sodium 109mg.

93 calories

Mini ciabatta pizzas

Most kids love pizzas, but store-bought ones tend to be high in fat, salt and calories. These home-made ones are much healthier, and you can adapt the toppings to suit.

serves 8

2 red and 2 yellow (bell) peppers
1 loaf ciabatta bread
8 slices prosciutto
150g/5oz reduced-fat mozzarella cheese
ground black pepper, to taste
tiny basil leaves, to garnish

1 Preheat a grill (broiler). Halve the peppers and remove their seeds. Place the peppers on a grill rack. Grill (broil) until the outsides are beginning to turn black.

2 Place the charred peppers in a bowl, cover with clear film or plastic wrap and leave to sweat for 10 minutes.

3 Meanwhile, cut the bread into eight thick slices and toast both sides under the grill until golden. Leave the grill on.

4 Peel off the skins from the peppers (sweating will have loosened them). Cut both the peppers and the prosciutto into thick strips and arrange these on the toasted bread.

5 Slice the mozzarella cheese and arrange it on top. Grind over black pepper to taste. Place the bread slices back under the grill and cook for 2–3 minutes, until the cheese is bubbling.

6 Remove the pizzas from the grill. Arrange the fresh basil leaves on top and serve the pizzas immediately, or leave them to cool completely and then wrap in clear film or plastic wrap to transport for lunch.

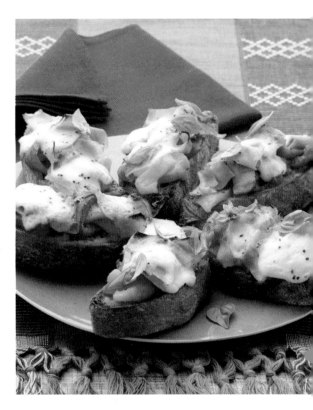

variations

• For speed, you could use 4 drained bottled roasted (bell) peppers instead of grilling (broiling) your own. Alternatively, if the children like raw pepper, just dice some and use it raw.
• You can try all sorts of toppings on this pizza: corn or chopped tomato are especially popular.

Per portion Energy 227kcal/958kJ; Protein 11.8g; Carbohydrate 31.6g, of which sugars 6.9g; Fat 6.8g, of which saturates 3g; Cholesterol 9mg; Calcium 124mg; Fibre 3.5g; Sodium 547mg.

227
calories

Roast tomato pasta salad

Pasta salads are great for packed lunches, as they are very portable and sustaining as well as being low in fat. This one contains roasted tomatoes, which are sweet, tender and juicy, especially when tomatoes are out of season. During the summer, you could just use ripe raw tomatoes for speed, if you prefer.

serves 4

450g/1lb ripe baby Italian plum tomatoes
45ml/3 tbsp extra virgin olive oil
2 garlic cloves, peeled and cut into thin slivers
a pinch of salt
225g/8oz/2 cups dried pasta shapes, preferably
    wholemeal (whole-wheat), such as shells,
    butterflies or spirals
30ml/2 tbsp balsamic vinegar
2 sun-dried tomatoes in olive oil,
    drained and chopped
a pinch of sugar
ground black pepper, to taste
1 handful rocket (arugula)

1 Cut the tomatoes in half lengthways. Arrange, cut-side up, in a roasting pan. Drizzle 30ml/2 tbsp of the olive oil over them and sprinkle with the slivers of garlic. Season with a pinch of salt to draw out the juices.

2 Preheat the oven to 190°C/375°F/Gas 5.

3 Place the tomatoes in the preheated oven and roast for about 20 minutes, turning once, until they are soft and the skin is turning golden. Set aside to cool.

4 Halfway through the cooking time in step 3, two-thirds fill a large pan with water. Bring to the boil. Add the pasta and bring back to the boil. Cook for 8–10 minutes, or according to packet instructions, until just tender (al dente).

5 Put the remaining oil in a bowl with the vinegar, sun-dried tomatoes, sugar and a little pepper to taste. Stir to mix.

6 Drain the pasta and add it to the bowl of dressing and toss to mix. Add the roasted tomatoes and mix gently.

7 Before serving, add the rocket leaves and toss gently to combine. Serve warm or leave until cool, then chill. To transport, pack into a sealable plastic container.

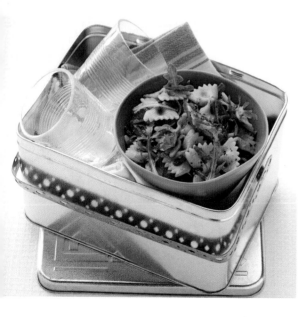

Per portion Energy 361kcal/1518kJ; Protein 8.2g; Carbohydrate 46g, of which sugars 5.9g; Fat 17.3g, of which saturates 2.4g; Cholesterol 0mg; Calcium 43mg; Fibre 4g; Sodium 151mg.

361 calories

Chicken pasta salad

Packed with colourful, crunchy veg and succulent chunks of cold roast chicken, this scrummy salad is perfect for using up Sunday's leftover chicken. You could also use cooked turkey or some drained canned salmon. For a vegetarian version, omit the chicken and Worcestershire sauce and include some chopped hard-boiled eggs.

serves 6

350g/12oz dried pasta shapes, preferably
  wholemeal (whole-wheat)
30ml/2 tbsp olive oil
225g/8oz cold cooked chicken
2 small red or yellow (bell) peppers
4 spring onions (scallions)
50g/2oz/⅓ cup pitted green olives
45ml/3 tbsp low-fat mayonnaise
5ml/1 tsp Worcestershire sauce
5ml/1 tsp wine vinegar
ground black pepper, to taste
fresh basil leaves, to garnish

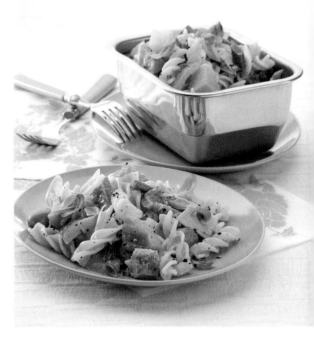

1 Two-thirds fill a large pan with water. Bring to the boil. Add the pasta and bring back to the boil. Cook for 8–10 minutes, or according to the packet instructions, until just tender (al dente).

2 Drain and rinse the pasta and put it in a large bowl. Toss with the olive oil to prevent it from sticking together.

3 Remove any bones, fat or skin from the chicken and cut the meat into bitesize pieces. Add to the bowl of pasta.

4 Seed the peppers, then chop them into pieces. Trim and slice the spring onions.

5 To the bowl of pasta add the pepper and spring onion along with all the remaining ingredients (except the basil). Season to taste with black pepper and mix to combine thoroughly.

6 Garnish with basil to serve, or pack into a sealable plastic container to transport.

cook's tip

• The pasta salad should be kept in a refrigerator if possible, especially during hot weather. Alternatively, use an insulated cool bag and include an ice pack to keep everything cool.

Per portion Energy 333kcal/1405kJ; Protein 19g; Carbohydrate 46.3g, of which sugars 4.6g; Fat 9.3g, of which saturates 1.5g; Cholesterol 32mg; Calcium 29mg; Fibre 3.4g; Sodium 294mg.

333 calories

Tuna and bean salad

It's worth keeping some cans of tuna and different types of beans handy in your storecupboard or pantry so that you can throw this together for a last-minute picnic.

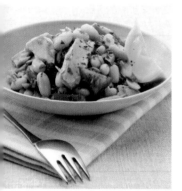

serves 4
. . . .

400g/14oz can
   cannellini beans
200g/7oz can tuna fish
   in spring water
15ml/1 tbsp olive oil
15ml/1 tbsp lemon juice
ground black pepper
10ml/2 tsp chopped
   fresh parsley
4 ripe tomatoes

1 Pour the canned beans into a colander and rinse well under plenty of cold running water. Drain well. Place in large serving dish.

2 Drain the tuna, put it in a medium bowl and break it into fairly large flakes with a fork. Arrange over the beans in the dish.

3 Make the dressing by combining the oil with the lemon juice in a small bowl. Season with pepper and stir in the parsley. Mix well.

4 Cut the tomatoes into chunks and add to the beans and tuna. Pour over the dressing and toss the mixture gently with a fork.

5 Serve immediately or chill until needed. To transport, pack into a well-sealed plastic container.

Per portion Energy 166kcal/704kJ; Protein 17.6g; Carbohydrate 16.5g, of which sugars 5.8g; Fat 3.8g, of which saturates 0.7g; Cholesterol 26mg; Calcium 64mg; Fibre 7.5g; Sodium 462mg.

166 calories

Lemony couscous salad

Couscous is a lovely light and fluffy grain that is perfect for making salads as it absorbs all of the delicious flavours. It makes a really quick lunchbox treat.

serves 4
. . . .

450ml/¾ pint/scant 2 cups low-salt vegetable stock
275g/10oz/1⅔ cups couscous
2 small courgettes (zucchini)
16–20 black olives, pitted and halved
25g/1oz/¼ cup flaked (sliced) almonds, toasted

for the dressing
60ml/4 tbsp olive oil
15ml/1 tbsp lemon juice
15ml/1 tbsp chopped fresh coriander (cilantro)
15ml/1 tbsp chopped fresh parsley
a pinch of ground cumin
a pinch of cayenne pepper

1 Put the stock into a pan and bring it to the boil. Place the couscous in a large heatproof bowl. Pour over the stock. Stir the couscous with a fork, then set aside for 10 minutes until the stock has been absorbed and the couscous is cooked.

2 Meanwhile, trim the courgettes and cut them into pieces about 2.5cm/1in long. Slice into strips.

3 Whisk together the dressing ingredients in a small bowl.

4 Fluff up the couscous with a fork, then mix in the dressing, courgette, olives and flaked almonds. Serve or pack into a plastic container.

Per portion Energy 336kcal/1392kJ; Protein 6.4g; Carbohydrate 37.6g, of which sugars 1.1g; Fat 18.6g, of which saturates 2.4g; Cholesterol 0mg; Calcium 60mg; Fibre 1.7g; Sodium 565mg.

336 calories

Confetti salad

This salad gets its name from the little pieces of brightly coloured diced vegetables that are mixed in with cold rice. You could add some chopped hard-boiled egg, drained fish such as tuna or salmon, or strips of roast chicken or turkey for protein. It is perfect for a tasty meal on the go.

serves 6

275g/10oz/1½ cups long grain rice
225g/8oz ripe tomatoes
1 green and 1 yellow (bell) pepper
1 bunch of spring onions (scallions)
30ml/2 tbsp chopped fresh flat leaf parsley
  or fresh coriander (cilantro)

for the dressing
75ml/5 tbsp olive oil
15ml/1 tbsp sherry vinegar
5ml/1 tsp Dijon mustard
salt and ground black pepper, to taste

1 Place the rice in a pan and cover with water. Bring to the boil and cook for 10–12 minutes, or according to packet instructions, until tender.

2 Drain the rice, then rinse and drain again. Leave to cool.

3 Meanwhile, place the tomatoes in a heatproof bowl and pour boiling water from the kettle over them to cover. Leave for 30 seconds or until the skins soften and start to split (if they don't split, pierce them with the tip of a sharp knife and they should start to split).

4 Drain the tomatoes in a colander, cool slightly, then peel away the skin with your fingers.

5 On a chopping board, cut the tomatoes into quarters. Carefully cut out the seeds and discard. Chop into chunks.

6 Cut the peppers in half. Cut out and discard the seeds and membranes. Dice the peppers. Trim and slice the spring onions.

7 To make the dressing, whisk all the ingredients together in a small bowl.

8 Transfer the rice to a large serving bowl with the tomatoes, peppers and spring onions. Add the herbs and the dressing. Mix well.

9 Serve, or chill until required. To transport, pack into a sealable plastic container.

Per portion Energy 276kcal/1150kJ; Protein 4.6g; Carbohydrate 41.9g, of which sugars 5.2g; Fat 9.9g, of which saturates 1.4g; Cholesterol 0mg; Calcium 29mg; Fibre 1.7g; Sodium 8mg.

276 calories

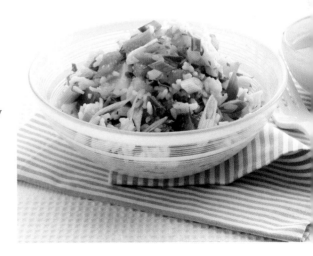

SOUPS AND SNACKS

Carrot soup

Carrots are packed with vitamins and minerals, and most children like their sweet flavour. The addition of lentils makes the soup more substantial, as well as adding protein and nutrients, and also gives it a lovely creamy texture once it is blended. Serve with toast or chunks of wholemeal (whole-wheat) bread for a healthy meal.

serves 6

450g/1lb carrots
1 onion
15ml/1 tbsp sunflower oil
75g/3oz/scant ½ cup split red lentils
1.2 litres/2 pints/5 cups low-salt vegetable or
    chicken stock
5ml/1 tsp ground coriander
45ml/3 tbsp chopped fresh parsley
salt and ground black pepper, to taste
fresh coriander (cilantro) leaves and low-fat natural
    (plain) yogurt, to serve

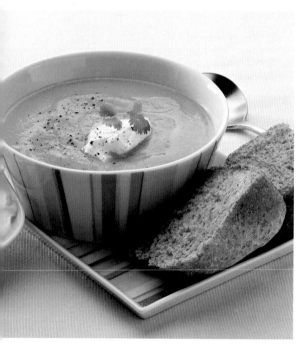

1 Peel the carrots, then trim off the ends and slice them into rounds. Peel the onion and cut it in half. Lay the halves flat and slice them into half-moon crescents.

2 Heat the oil in a pan, add the onion crescents and cook, stirring, for 5 minutes. Add the carrot rounds and cook gently, stirring, for 4–5 minutes, until they start to soften.

3 Meanwhile, put the lentils in a small bowl and cover with cold water. Skim off any bits that float on the surface. Tip into a fine strainer and rinse under cold running water.

4 Add the lentils, stock and ground coriander to the pan. Bring to the boil. Lower the heat, cover and simmer for 30 minutes, or until the lentils are tender.

5 Add the parsley, season to taste and cook for about 5 minutes. Set the pan aside and leave the mixture to cool slightly.

6 Pour the soup into a blender or food processor and blend until smooth. (You may have to do this in two batches.)

7 Return the soup to the pan and reheat until piping hot. Ladle into bowls and garnish with coriander and a spoonful of yogurt.

Per portion Energy 108kcal/449kJ; Protein 4g; Carbohydrate 16.9g, of which sugars 7.5g; Fat 3.1g, of which saturates 0.5g; Cholesterol 0mg; Calcium 36mg; Fibre 3.9g; Sodium 25mg.

108
calories

Broccoli soup

They call broccoli a superfood because it is packed with goodness. This soup is also full of flavour. Serve it with wholemeal bread for a satisfying lunch.

serves 6

675g/1½lb broccoli spears
1.75 litres/3 pints/7½ cups low-salt chicken stock
ground black pepper, to taste
30ml/1 tbsp fresh lemon juice
wholemeal (whole-wheat) bread, to serve (optional)

1 Using a vegetable peeler, peel the broccoli stems, starting from the base of the stalks and pulling up towards the florets. Chop the broccoli into small chunks.

2 Pour the stock into a large pan and bring to the boil. Add the broccoli. Simmer for 20 minutes, or until soft. Remove from the heat and cool.

3 Carefully pour half the mixture into a blender and blend until smooth. Stir this into the mixture in the pan. Season to taste and add lemon juice.

4 Serve the soup hot with bread, if you like.

cook's tip

• Frozen broccoli is ideal for this soup, and makes a cheap standby that is as packed with goodness as the fresh version. There is no need to defrost it before use, simply increase the cooking time if necessary, until the broccoli is cooked and soft enough to blend to a smooth soup.

Per portion Energy 61kcal/247kJ; Protein 5.3g; Carbohydrate 4.9g, of which sugars 2g; Fat 2.2g, of which saturates 0.5g; Cholesterol 0mg; Calcium 63mg; Fibre 3.9g; Sodium 9mg.

61 calories

Super-duper soup

This fantastic vegetable soup is healthy, tasty and extremely easy to make. You can vary the vegetables, using whichever ones you like best.

serves 6

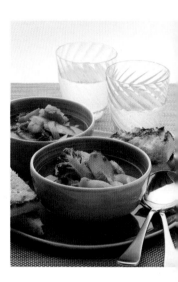

1 onion
2 carrots
675g/1½lb potatoes
115g/4oz broccoli
1 courgette (zucchini)
115g/4oz mushrooms
15ml/1 tbsp oil
1.2 litres/2 pints/5 cups
   low-salt stock
450g/1lb can
   chopped tomatoes
5ml/1 tsp dried herbs
ground black pepper,
   to taste

1 Peel the onion, carrots and potatoes. Slice the onion and carrots and cut the potatoes into large chunks. Cut the broccoli into florets. Slice the courgette and the mushrooms. Set aside.

2 Heat the oil in a pan. Add the onion and carrots and fry gently for about 10 minutes, stirring occasionally, until they soften.

3 Add the potatoes and fry for 2 minutes more, stirring. Add the remaining ingredients and bring to the boil. Cover the pan and simmer the mixture for 30–40 minutes, or until the vegetables are tender. Serve immediately.

Per portion Energy 152kcal/638kJ; Protein 4.7g; Carbohydrate 27g, of which sugars 7.4g; Fat 3.5g, of which saturates 0.6g; Cholesterol 37mg; Calcium 52mg; Fibre 4.4g; Sodium 52mg.

152 calories

Lentil soup

Red lentils and vegetables are cooked and puréed to make a smooth and very nutritious soup that kids will love. It freezes very well, so make double.

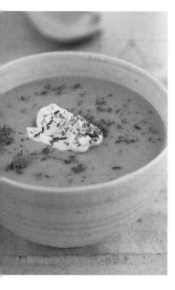

serves 6

45ml/3 tbsp olive oil
1 onion, peeled and
    chopped
2 celery sticks, chopped
2 carrots, chopped
2 garlic cloves, chopped
250g/9oz/generous
    1 cup red lentils, rinsed
1 litre/1¾ pints/4 cups
    low-salt stock
ground black pepper
low-fat natural (plain)
    yogurt, to serve
ground cumin,
    to serve

1 Heat the oil in a large pan. Add the onion and cook for about 10 minutes or until softened. Stir in the celery, carrots and garlic. Cook for a few minutes until beginning to soften.

2 Add the lentils and stock and bring to the boil. Reduce the heat, cover and simmer for about 30 minutes, until the lentils are tender.

3 Pour the soup into a food processor or blender and process until smooth. Tip the soup back into the pan and stir in the pepper. Ladle into bowls and top with some yogurt and ground cumin.

Per portion Energy 209kcal/876kJ; Protein 10.5g; Carbohydrate 28.1g, of which sugars 3.5g; Fat 6.8g, of which saturates 1.1g; Cholesterol 0mg; Calcium 35mg; Fibre 3.7g; Sodium 25mg.

209 calories

Corn and potato chowder

This creamy, chunky soup is rich with the sweet taste of corn and is very nutritious. It makes a warming meal-in-a-bowl and requires no accompaniment.

serves 4

1 onion, peeled and chopped
1 garlic clove, peeled and crushed
1 medium baking potato, peeled and chopped
2 celery sticks, chopped
1 small green (bell) pepper, seeded and chopped
30ml/2 tbsp sunflower oil
25g/1oz/2 tbsp unsalted butter
600ml/1 pint/2½ cups low-salt stock or water
ground black pepper, to taste
300ml/½ pint/1¼ cups semi-skimmed (low-fat) milk
200g/7oz can cannellini beans
300g/11oz can corn
a good pinch of dried sage

1 Put the onion, garlic, potato, celery and pepper into a large heavy pan with the oil and butter.

2 Heat over a medium heat until sizzling, then reduce the heat to low. Cover and cook for about 10 minutes, stirring occasionally, until the vegetables have softened slightly.

3 Pour in the stock or water, season and bring to the boil. Reduce the heat, cover and simmer for about 15 minutes, until the vegetables are tender.

4 Add the milk, beans and corn – with their liquids – and the sage. Simmer, uncovered, for 5 minutes. Serve.

Per portion Energy 313kcal/1314kJ; Protein 10.6g; Carbohydrate 37.8g, of which sugars 9.8g; Fat 14.4g, of which saturates 5.2g; Cholesterol 35mg; Calcium 124mg; Fibre 7.9g; Sodium 95mg.

313 calories

Tomato and bread soup

This simple tomato and basil soup is thickened with stale bread, making it thrifty as well as nutritious and sustaining. It can be made all year round, since you can use canned tomatoes in place of fresh ones during the winter months. For a lower-fat version, simply toast rather than frying the bread, before cutting it into chunks.

serves 6

175g/6oz stale bread, preferably wholemeal
   (whole-wheat)
1 medium onion
2 garlic cloves
45ml/3 tbsp olive oil
675g/1½lb ripe tomatoes, peeled and chopped,
   or 2 x 400g/14oz cans plum tomatoes, chopped
45ml/3 tbsp chopped fresh basil
ground black pepper, to taste
1.5 litres/2½ pints/6¼ cups low-salt vegetable
   stock or water, or a combination
fresh basil leaves, to garnish

1 Cut away the crusts from the bread using a large serrated knife. Cut into cubes. Peel and finely chop the onion and garlic.

2 Heat 30ml/2 tbsp of the oil in a large pan. Add the bread cubes and cook, stirring, until golden in colour. Remove with a slotted spoon and transfer to a plate lined with kitchen paper. Set aside.

3 Add the remaining oil along with the onion and garlic to the pan and cook, stirring often, for about 10 minutes or until the onion softens.

4 Stir in the tomatoes, bread cubes and chopped basil. Season to taste with pepper. Cook over a moderate heat, stirring occasionally, for 15 minutes.

5 Meanwhile, place the stock or water in a pan and bring to a boil.

6 Add the boiling stock and/or water to the pan containing the tomato mixture and mix well. Bring to a boil, lower the heat slightly and simmer for 20 minutes.

7 Remove the soup from the heat. Use a fork to mash the tomatoes and the bread together.

8 Allow the soup to stand for 10 minutes before serving, garnished with basil leaves.

Per portion Energy 165kcal/690kJ; Protein 4g; Carbohydrate 22.2g, of which sugars 5.9g; Fat 7.3g, of which saturates 1.2g; Cholesterol 0mg; Calcium 65mg; Fibre 2.6g; Sodium 163mg.

165 calories

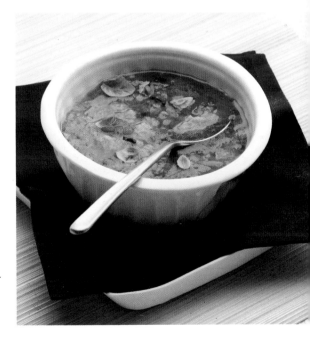

Chinese chicken soup

You may have had something similar to this delicious meal-in-a-bowl soup in a restaurant before, but this home-made version wins hands-down for taste.

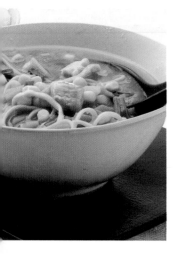

serves 6

225g/8oz chicken
   breast fillets
15ml/1 tbsp oil
4 spring onions
   (scallions), chopped
1.2 litres/2 pints/5 cups
   low-salt chicken stock
5ml/1 tsp soy sauce
115g/4oz/1 cup
   frozen corn
115g/4oz medium
   egg noodles
1 carrot, thinly sliced

1 Remove the skin from the chicken, then trim off any fat and cut the meat into small cubes.

2 Heat the oil in a pan. Add the chicken and onions. Cook, stirring, until the meat is browned. Add the stock and soy sauce and bring to the boil.

3 Stir in the corn, then add the egg noodles, breaking them up roughly with your fingers.

4 Simmer, uncovered, for 1–2 minutes until the noodles and corn are beginning to soften. Add the carrot and simmer for 5 minutes.

5 Ladle into bowls and serve immediately.

Per portion Energy 172kcal/722kJ; Protein 12.5g; Carbohydrate 20.4g, of which sugars 2.3g; Fat 5g, of which saturates 1.1g; Cholesterol 32mg; Calcium 14mg; Fibre 1.7g; Sodium 239mg.

172
calories

Chicken and leek soup

This makes a substantial main course soup when served with bread. It takes a while to cook, but the recipe makes a lot, so freeze some for another time.

serves 8

1.4kg/3lb chicken pieces
1 small head of celery, trimmed
1 onion, peeled and coarsely chopped
1 fresh bay leaf
a few fresh parsley stalks
a few fresh tarragon sprigs
2.4 litres/4 pints/10 cups cold water
65g/2½oz/5 tbsp unsalted butter
3 large leeks, sliced
2 potatoes, peeled and cut into chunks
salt and ground black pepper, to taste

1 To make the stock, put the chicken into a large pan with half the celery and the onion. Tie the bay leaf, parsley and tarragon together and add to the pan with the water and bring to the boil. Reduce heat, cover and simmer for 1½ hours.

2 Remove the chicken and cut off, chop up and reserve the meat (discard the skin, bones and gristle). Strain the stock, then return it to the pan and boil until it has reduced to 1.5 litres/2½ pints/6¼ cups.

3 Melt the butter in a large pan. Add the leeks and remaining celery, cover and cook over a low heat for 10 minutes. Add the potatoes and stock. Season, part-cover the pan and simmer until the potatoes are cooked. Add the chopped chicken, then process the soup until smooth. Reheat if necessary and serve.

Per portion Energy 256kcal/1075kJ; Protein 30.5g; Carbohydrate 10.4g, of which sugars 2.5g; Fat 10.6g, of which saturates 5.3g; Cholesterol 111mg; Calcium 36mg; Fibre 3.1g; Sodium 124mg.

256
calories

Beef broth with vegetables

Good beef stock is an essential base for this soup. When home-made stock is not available, use a high-quality, low-salt chilled commercial one, rather than a stock cube. Since Parmesan has a lovely strong flavour, only a little is required, but you could leave it off if you prefer.

serves 6

45ml/3 tbsp vegetable oil
1 onion, peeled and chopped
2 garlic cloves, peeled and finely chopped
2 carrots, peeled and diced
1 leek, thinly sliced
a large pinch of saffron threads
150g/5oz/¾ cup long grain rice
2 litres/3½ pints/8 cups low-salt beef stock
½ butternut squash, diced
2 medium potatoes, peeled and diced
100g/4oz/1 cup frozen peas, thawed
ground black pepper, to taste
a little freshly grated Parmesan cheese,
   to serve (optional)

1 Heat the vegetable oil in a large pan, add the onion and cook gently for 10 minutes, or until it is softened.

2 Add the garlic and cook gently for a further 2 minutes. Add the carrots, leek and saffron and cook for 2–3 minutes, stirring frequently.

3 Sprinkle over the rice and stir for a minute to coat in the juices, then pour in the stock. Bring to the boil, lower the heat and cover the pan with a lid. Simmer for 10 minutes.

4 Add the diced squash and potatoes, then re-cover the pan and simmer for 15 minutes more or until the vegetables and rice are tender. Stir in the peas and season to taste with ground black pepper.

5 Bring to the boil and cook for 1 minute, then cover the pan with a lid and leave to stand for a few minutes before serving.

6 Ladle into warmed bowls and sprinkle with grated Parmesan, if using.

Per portion Energy 290kcal/1207kJ; Protein 6.3g; Carbohydrate 46.9g, of which sugars 8.9g; Fat 9.1g, of which saturates 4.9g; Cholesterol 40mg; Calcium 69mg; Fibre 5.7g; Sodium 69mg.

290 calories

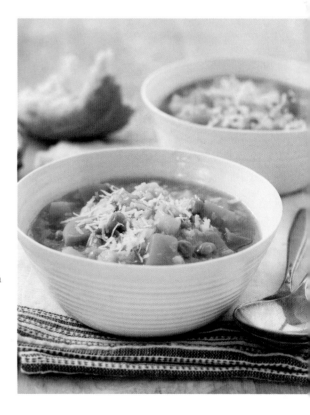

Crunchy veggie salad

This crunchy snack is packed with vitamins and will give children loads of energy – ideal for after school, to get them through their homework. Serve it with slices of wholemeal bread, or pack it up in a container to take to school or on a picnic. If they don't like one particular ingredient, swap it for something else.

serves 4–6
. . . .

¼ small white cabbage
¼ small red cabbage
8 baby carrots
50g/2oz small mushrooms
115g/4oz cauliflower
1 small courgette (zucchini)
10cm/4in piece cucumber
2 tomatoes
50g/2oz sprouted seeds (see cook's tip)
50g/2oz/½ cup peanuts (optional)
30ml/2 tbsp sunflower oil
15ml/1 tbsp lemon juice
ground black pepper, to taste
50g/2oz low-fat hard cheese

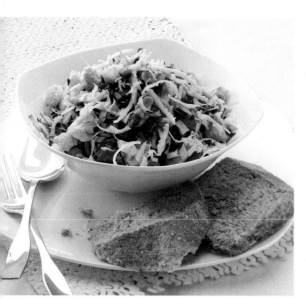

1 On a chopping board, finely chop the white and red cabbage. Peel the carrots, then slice them into thin rounds or sticks.

2 Gently wipe the mushrooms clean, then cut them into quarters. Cut the cauliflower into small, even-size florets.

3 Grate the courgette with a coarse grater. Cut the cucumber into cubes and chop the tomatoes into similar-size pieces.

4 Put all the prepared vegetables and sprouted seeds in a bowl and mix together well.

5 Stir in the peanuts, if using. Drizzle over the oil and lemon juice. Season well and leave to stand for 30 minutes to allow the flavours to develop.

6 Grate the cheese coarsely and sprinkle over just before serving with slices of crusty bread.

cook's tip
. . . .

• Sprouted seeds are seeds (typically mung beans or soy beans) that, under the right conditions, have started to grow shoots. They taste great and are full of goodness. You can either buy them from a supermarket, or you could try sprouting your own at home. It is very easy: all you need is some damp kitchen paper and the right seeds.

Per portion Energy 99kcal/410kJ; Protein 5.1g; Carbohydrate 7g, of which sugars 6.3g; Fat 5.7g, of which saturates 1.4g; Cholesterol 4mg; Calcium 138mg; Fibre 4.9g; Sodium 83mg.

99 calories

Chicken and tomato salad

Warm salads are lovely for eating all year round but especially in winter when you fancy a salad but need warm food. This one is delicious and nutritious.

serves 2

225g/8oz baby spinach leaves, rinsed and trimmed
250g/9oz cherry tomatoes, halved
½ bunch spring onions (scallions), finely chopped
1 large skinless chicken breast fillet
ground black pepper, to taste

for the dressing
45ml/3 tbsp olive oil
15ml/1 tbsp hazelnut oil
5ml/1 tbsp white wine vinegar
1 garlic clove, peeled and crushed
15ml/1 tbsp chopped fresh mixed herbs

1 To make the dressing, whisk together 30ml/ 2 tbsp of the olive oil and the hazelnut oil, then slowly add the vinegar, whisking well between each addition. Add the crushed garlic and chopped mixed herbs and whisk to combine.

2 Put the spinach, tomatoes and spring onion in a large serving bowl.

3 Cut the chicken into thin strips. Heat the remaining olive oil in a frying pan and stir-fry the chicken over a high heat for 7–10 minutes, until it is cooked and brown. Arrange over the salad.

4 Drizzle over the dressing, season to taste, toss lightly and serve immediately.

Per portion Energy 322kcal/1339kJ; Protein 27.5g; Carbohydrate 6.6g, of which sugars 6.4g; Fat 20.8g, of which saturates 3.4g; Cholesterol 62mg; Calcium 224mg; Fibre 5.5g; Sodium 221mg.

322 calories

Summer rolls

These rolls are crunchy and pretty as well as tasty – perfect for a quick light meal in the summer. Older children in particular will enjoy assembling and eating these.

serves 6

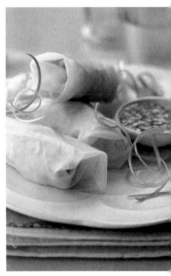

12 round rice papers
12 lettuce leaves
1 small cucumber, peeled, seeded and cut into fine strips
2–3 carrots, peeled and cut into fine strips
3 spring onions (scallions), cut into fine strips
225g/8oz beansprouts
1 bunch of mint leaves
1 bunch of fresh coriander (cilantro)
low-sugar Asian dipping sauce, to serve

1 Pour some lukewarm water into a shallow dish. Soak the rice papers, two or three at a time, for 5 minutes, until soft. Place on a dish towel; cover.

2 Work with one paper at a time. Place a lettuce leaf towards the edge nearest to you, leaving 2.5cm/ 1in to fold over. Place a mixture of the vegetables on top, followed by some mint and coriander.

3 Fold the edge nearest to you over the filling, tuck in the sides, and roll tightly to the edge on the far side. Repeat with the other papers and vegetables. Serve with dipping sauce.

Per portion Energy 106Kcal/445kJ; Protein 3.5g; Carbohydrate 21.2g, of which sugars 4.7g; Fat 0.7g, of which saturates 0.2g; Cholesterol 0mg; Calcium 44mg; Fibre 2.2g; Sodium 10mg.

106 calories

Tortilla squares

Spanish omelette, or tortilla, makes a great supper, but if you cut it into small squares you can enjoy it as a 'nibble' at parties or just as a healthy snack. Try serving the pieces on cocktail sticks or toothpicks and accompanying it with wholemeal bread, olives, roasted peppers and some dips for a tapas-style supper.

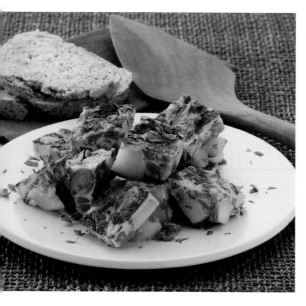

serves 8 as a snack or 4 as a main

45ml/3 tbsp olive oil
2 Spanish (Bermuda) onions, peeled and sliced
300g/11oz waxy potatoes, cut into 1cm/½in dice
250g/9oz/1¾ cups shelled broad (fava) beans
5ml/1 tsp chopped fresh thyme
salt and ground black pepper, to taste
6 large (US extra-large) eggs
45ml/3 tbsp chopped fresh chives and parsley

1 Heat 30ml/2 tbsp of the oil in a deep 23cm/9in non-stick frying pan. Add the onions and potatoes and stir to coat. Cover and cook, stirring frequently, for 20–25 minutes, until the potatoes are cooked and the onions are very soft.

2 Meanwhile, two-thirds fill a medium pan with cold water. Bring to the boil. Add the beans and cook for 3 minutes, until tender. Drain them well and put in a large bowl to cool.

3 When the beans are cool enough to handle, peel off and discard the grey outer skins. This is quite fussy, but fun, so get the kids involved with this stage.

4 Add the beans and thyme to the onions and potatoes in the frying pan. Season, stir well to mix, then cook for a further 2–3 minutes.

5 Beat the eggs and fresh herbs in a bowl. Add to the pan and increase the heat.

6 Cook until the egg browns underneath, pulling it away from the sides of the pan and tilting it to allow the uncooked egg to run underneath.

7 Cover the pan with an upside-down plate and invert the tortilla on to it.

8 Heat the remaining oil in the pan. Slip the tortilla back into the pan, uncooked-side down, and cook for 3–5 minutes more, until brown.

9 Slide the tortilla on to a serving plate. Cut it into squares if serving it as a snack or cut it into quarters and serve with salad as a light meal.

Per portion (8) Energy 177kcal/738kJ; Protein 9.2g; Carbohydrate 15.5g, of which sugars 4.8g; Fat 9.2g, of which saturates 1.9g; Cholesterol 150mg; Calcium 71mg; Fibre 3.7g; Sodium 66mg.

177
calories

Chicken mini rolls

These small, crispy rolls can be served warm for a party buffet or as a snack. If you want to get ahead, make them the day before, then reheat in the oven. Filo pastry is much lower in fat than other types, and lean chicken makes a healthy filling. You could use turkey or pork instead if you want to ring the changes.

makes about 10

1 x 275g/10oz packet filo pastry, thawed if frozen
45ml/3 tbsp olive oil, for brushing

for the filling
350g/12oz minced (ground) chicken,
1 egg, beaten
2.5ml/½ tsp ground cinnamon
2.5ml/½ tsp ground ginger
30ml/2 tbsp raisins
ground black pepper, to taste
15ml/1 tbsp olive oil
1 small onion, peeled and finely chopped

1 First, make the filling. Put the minced chicken, beaten egg, cinnamon, ginger and raisins in a large mixing bowl and season well with ground black pepper.

2 Gently heat the oil in a frying pan, add the chopped onion and cook over a low heat, stirring occasionally, for 10 minutes, until tender. Leave to cool, then add to the bowl.

3 Preheat the oven to 180°C/350°F/Gas 4. Line a baking sheet with baking parchment. Open the filo pastry and unravel. Cut the pastry into 10 x 25cm/4 x 10in strips.

4 Take one strip of pastry, keeping the remainder covered, and brush with oil. Place a small spoonful of the filling about 1cm/½in from the end of the pastry strip.

5 Fold the sides inwards to a width of 5cm/2in and roll into a roll shape. Place the roll on the baking sheet and brush the top with oil. Repeat steps 4 and 5 with the remaining ingredients.

6 Bake for 20–25 minutes, until golden brown and crisp. Remove from the oven and transfer to a wire rack. Serve hot or warm.

cook's tip

• Once filo pastry is exposed it dries out fast, so it is important to work quickly once the pastry is opened and keep any you are not using covered with clear film or plastic wrap.

Per portion Energy 158kcal/663kJ; Protein 10.9g; Carbohydrate 16.9g, of which sugars 2.7g; Fat 5.6g, of which saturates 0.9g; Cholesterol 44mg; Calcium 40mg; Fibre 1g; Sodium 31mg.

158 calories

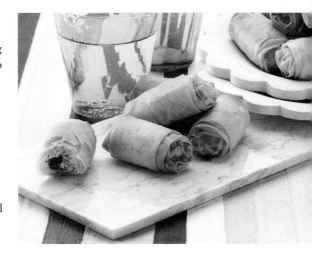

MAIN MEALS

Quick and easy risotto

A traditional Italian risotto is made by gradually stirring stock into rice as it cooks. This recipe is a cheats' dish because it all goes in the pan at the same time.

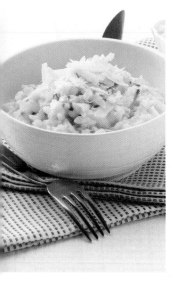

serves 4

75g/3oz sliced good-
  quality cooked ham,
  chicken or turkey
1 litre/1¾ pints/4 cups
  low-salt chicken
  stock
275g/10oz/1½ cups
  risotto rice
30ml/2 tbsp freshly
  grated Parmesan
30ml/2 tbsp roughly
  chopped fresh
  parsley leaves
ground black pepper,
  to taste

1 Cut the ham, chicken or turkey into similar-size squares.

2 Put the stock in a large pan and bring to the boil. Reduce the heat and add the rice. Bring back to the boil. Cover and simmer, stirring regularly, for 18–20 minutes, until the rice is tender.

3 Remove from the heat and stir in the Parmesan, cooked meat and parsley. Season to taste with pepper. Cover the pan and leave to stand for 2–3 minutes, then stir again to combine thoroughly. Serve the risotto immediately.

Per portion Energy 325kcal/1354kJ; Protein 12.3g; Carbohydrate 57.7g, of which sugars 0.6g; Fat 4.6g, of which saturates 2g; Cholesterol 18mg; Calcium 106mg; Fibre 0.5g; Sodium 256mg.

325 calories

Mexican tomato rice

This dish is a delicious mixture of rice, tomatoes, peas and spices. If your family doesn't like too much heat, reduce the number of chillies you use, or omit them.

serves 4

400g/14oz can chopped tomatoes
30ml/2 tbsp olive oil
½ onion, peeled and roughly chopped
2 garlic cloves, peeled and chopped
500g/1¼lb/2½ cups long grain rice
750ml/1¼ pints/3 cups low-salt vegetable stock
2.5ml/½ tsp salt
1–2 fresh mild chillies (optional)
150g/5oz/1 cup frozen peas
ground black pepper, to taste

1 Blend the tomatoes and their juice until smooth.

2 Heat the oil in a pan. Add the onion and garlic and cook over a medium heat, stirring, for about 10 minutes, until softened.

3 Stir in the rice and fry for 1–2 minutes. Add the tomatoes and cook, stirring, for 3–4 minutes until the liquid has evaporated.

4 Stir in the stock, salt, chillies (if using) and peas. Bring to the boil. Cover and simmer for 6 minutes, until the rice is tender.

5 Remove from the heat, cover and leave to stand for 5 minutes, so the flavours are absorbed. Remove the chillies, fluff up the rice with a fork and serve, seasoned with ground black pepper.

Per portion Energy 566kcal/2360kJ; Protein 13.2g; Carbohydrate 110g, of which sugars 4.7g; Fat 7.6g, of which saturates 1.2g; Cholesterol 0mg; Calcium 48mg; Fibre 3.6g; Sodium 286mg.

566 calories

Vegetable paella

This extremely easy all-in-one-pan meal includes lots of colourful, tasty vegetables and is a sure hit with vegetarians and meat-eaters alike. You can easily adapt this basic recipe by adding seafood (see variation below), strips of cooked chicken or turkey, or even some stir-fried lean beef.

serves 6

2 leeks
3 celery sticks, including leaves
1 red (bell) pepper
2 courgettes (zucchini)
175g/6oz/2½ cups brown cap (cremini) mushrooms
15ml/1 tbsp olive oil
1 onion, peeled and chopped
2 garlic cloves, peeled and chopped
175g/6oz/1½ cups frozen peas
450g/1lb/2 cups long grain brown rice
900ml/1½ pints/3¾ cups low-salt vegetable stock
a few saffron threads (optional)
400g/14oz can cannellini beans, drained
225g/8oz/2 cups cherry tomatoes
45–60ml/3–4 tbsp chopped fresh herbs

1 Slice the leeks and chop the celery, reserving any leaves. Cut the pepper in half, remove and discard the seeds and membranes, and slice. Chop the courgettes and the mushrooms.

2 Heat the oil in a large frying pan. Add the onion, garlic, leeks and celery and fry for about 10 minutes, until softened.

3 Add the pepper, courgettes, mushrooms, peas, brown rice, vegetable stock and saffron threads (if using) and mix well to combine.

4 Bring the mixture to the boil, stirring often. Lower the heat and simmer, uncovered, stirring often, for 30 minutes, until almost all the liquid has been absorbed and the rice is tender.

5 Add the beans and cook for 5 minutes more.

6 Meanwhile, cut the cherry tomatoes in half and add to the pan with the herbs. Serve immediately, garnished with the reserved celery leaves.

variation

• For a fuss-free seafood version of this dish, thaw 400g/14oz frozen premium seafood selection and 115g/4oz frozen large tiger prawns (shrimp) and add them in step 5 in place of the beans.

Per portion Energy 406kcal/1700kJ; Protein 14.2g; Carbohydrate 81.2g, of which sugars 9.2g; Fat 2.8g, of which saturates 0.6g; Cholesterol 0mg; Calcium 103mg; Fibre 10.5g; Sodium 233mg.

406 calories

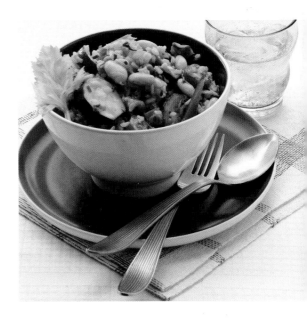

Popeye's pie

Popeye was a famous cartoon character who ate lots of spinach to make him really strong. Tuck into this crunchy layered pie at lunchtime and you too can have bulging muscles! Heart-healthy olive oil is used in place of butter to brush the pastry in this recipe.

serves 4

45ml/3 tbsp olive oil, plus extra for greasing
900g/2lb fresh spinach, stalks removed
50g/2oz low-fat Cheddar cheese, grated
115g/4oz/⅔ cup low-fat feta cheese, drained
ground black pepper, to taste
275g/10oz filo pastry
2.5ml/½ tsp each of ground cinnamon,
    ground nutmeg and ground black pepper

1 Preheat the oven to 160°C/325°F/Gas 3. Brush the inside of a roasting pan with a little oil.

2 Rinse the spinach in a colander, then tip it into a large pan. Cover and cook the spinach over a medium heat for 2–3 minutes, until it has wilted. Drain the spinach, leave it to cool, then squeeze it with your hands or press it with a clean dish towel to remove as much liquid as possible.

3 Put the Cheddar in a bowl, then crumble in the feta. Add some black pepper and stir to mix.

4 Unfold the pastry so the sheets are flat. Peel off a sheet and use to line part of the base of the roasting pan. Brush the pastry with oil. Keep the remaining sheets covered with a damp dish towel.

5 Continue to lay filo pastry sheets across the base and up the sides of the pan, brushing each time with oil, until two-thirds of the pastry has been used. Don't worry if the sheets flop over the top edges of the pan – they will be tidied up later.

6 Put the cool, squeezed spinach in a mixing bowl and break up any clumps with a fork. Add to the bowl containing the cheeses and combine.

7 Spoon the mixture into the pastry-lined pan and spread out. Fold the pastry edges over the filling.

8 Crumple up the remaining sheets of pastry and arrange them over the top of the filling. Brush the pastry with the remaining oil and sprinkle the mixed spices over the top.

9 Put in the oven and bake for 45 minutes. Raise the temperature to 200°C/400°F/Gas 6. Cook for 10–15 minutes more, until golden and crispy.

10 Remove from the oven and leave to cool in the pan for 5 minutes. Cut into squares and serve.

Per portion Energy 407kcal/1703kJ; Protein 19.8g; Carbohydrate 42.9g, of which sugars 4.6g; Fat 18.7g, of which saturates 6.7g; Cholesterol 26mg; Calcium 735mg; Fibre 8.4g; Sodium 816mg.

407
calories

Creamy coconut noodles

When everyday vegetables such as carrots and cabbage are given the Thai treatment, the result is a delectable creamy dish that everyone will enjoy. If your family likes their food spicy, you could add a little more red curry paste.

serves 4

30ml/2 tbsp vegetable oil
1 lemon grass stalk, finely chopped
15ml/1 tbsp Thai red curry paste
1 onion, peeled, halved and sliced
3 courgettes (zucchini), sliced into rounds
115g/4oz Savoy cabbage, shredded
2 carrots, peeled and sliced into rounds
150g/5oz broccoli, cut into florets
2 x 400ml/14fl oz cans reduced-fat coconut milk
475ml/16fl oz/2 cups low-salt vegetable stock
150g/5oz dried egg noodles
60ml/4 tbsp chopped fresh coriander (cilantro)
15ml/1 tbsp reduced-salt Thai fish sauce

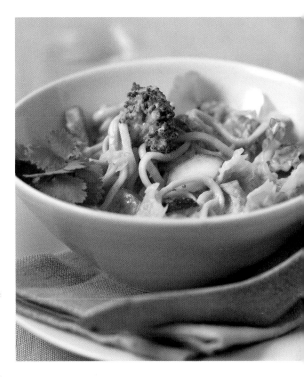

1 Heat the oil in a large pan or wok until just smoking. Add the lemon grass and red curry paste and stir-fry for 2–3 seconds, keeping it moving all the time.

2 Add the onion and reduce the heat to medium. Cook, stirring occasionally with a wooden spoon, for about 10 minutes, until the onion has softened but not browned.

3 Add the courgettes, cabbage, carrots and broccoli florets to the pan. Using two spoons, toss the vegetables to combine everything well. Reduce the heat to low.

4 Cook the mixture, stirring often, for a further 5 minutes, until the vegetables are softened. Increase the heat to medium, then stir in the coconut milk, stock and noodles and bring to the boil.

5 Add the coriander to the pan with the fish sauce. Stir and cook for 1 minute. Transfer to bowls and serve immediately.

cook's tip

• Many children enjoy spicy food, and this is fairly mild, so don't be afraid to give it to them to try. If they don't give it a go, they will never know!

Per portion Energy 326kcal/1366kJ; Protein 11.1g; Carbohydrate 46.5g, of which sugars 18.2g; Fat 11.8g, of which saturates 2.3g; Cholesterol 11mg; Calcium 179mg; Fibre 7.2g; Sodium 370mg.

326 calories

Presto pasta sauces

Pasta is an invaluable family food and it makes an appearance on most dinner tables several times a week. Although pasta itself isn't unhealthy (it is a great zero-fat carbohydrate), store-bought sauces can be very high in fat, salt and sugar, so it is much better to make your own and control what goes in them.

each serves 4–6

400g/14oz pasta

for the basic tomato sauce
15ml/1 tbsp olive oil
1 garlic clove, peeled and finely chopped
1 small onion, peeled and finely chopped
1 celery stick, finely chopped
400g/14oz can chopped tomatoes,
a handful fresh basil leaves, torn
ground black pepper, to taste

for the roasted vegetable sauce
2 red or orange (bell) peppers
1 small onion, peeled
1 small aubergine (eggplant)
2 tomatoes
2 garlic cloves, unpeeled
30ml/2 tbsp olive oil, to taste
15ml/1 tbsp lemon juice, to taste

for the pesto sauce
50g/2oz/1 cup basil leaves
1 garlic clove, peeled and finely chopped
30ml/2 tbsp pine nuts
ground black pepper, to taste
90ml/6 tbsp olive oil
30ml/2 tbsp freshly grated Parmesan cheese

for the nut cream sauce
115g/4oz/½ cup sugar-free no-salt smooth
   nut butter (such as almond or cashew nut)
a squeeze of lemon juice
ground black pepper, to taste

1 Make your chosen sauce, then cook the pasta in a large pan of boiling water for 8–10 minutes. In the case of the **nut cream sauce**: make it after cooking the pasta, using some reserved hot water.

2 To make the **basic tomato sauce**, heat the oil in a heavy pan. Add garlic, onion and celery. Cook over a low heat, stirring occasionally, for about 10–15 minutes until the onion softens and begins to colour.

3 Stir in the tomatoes and bring to the boil. Reduce the heat, cover and simmer for 10–15 minutes, stirring occasionally, until the mixture is thick.

4 Add the basil leaves, season with ground black pepper and stir. Serve hot with cooked pasta.

5 To make the **roasted vegetable sauce**, cut the peppers, onion, aubergine and tomatoes in half. Remove and discard any seeds and membranes from the various vegetables.

6 Preheat the grill (broiler). Place the vegetables on a baking sheet with the garlic.

7 Place under the grill and cook until the skins are blackened and charred, and the flesh is tender. Remove from the heat and leave until cool.

8 Peel the skins from the peppers, onions and tomatoes. Scoop the flesh from the aubergines and squeeze the flesh from the garlic.

9 Place the vegetables in a blender or food processor and blend to a smooth purée.

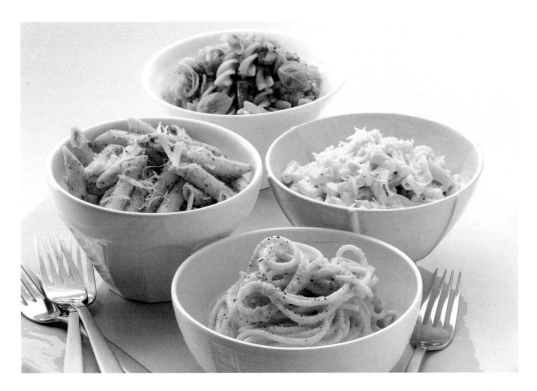

10 Taste, and add oil and lemon juice if necessary. If you prefer a smooth sauce, rub the purée through a sieve or strainer. Serve hot with cooked pasta.

11 To make the **pesto sauce**, place the basil, garlic, pine nuts and seasoning in a blender or food processor. Blend until smooth.

12 With the motor running, add the oil in a thin stream. Add the cheese and blend well.

13 Heat the sauce in a small pan. Serve hot with cooked pasta.

14 To make the **nut cream sauce**, put the nut butter in a bowl. Stir in a few tablespoons of the hot pasta cooking water and blend until smooth.

15 Gradually work in more hot water; up to 250ml/8fl oz/1 cup will make a thick sauce. Add lemon juice and seasoning to taste, then toss with cooked pasta.

Tomato sauce with pasta: per portion Energy 402kcal/1682kJ; Protein 0.8g; Carbohydrate 2.8g, of which sugars 2.5g; Fat 1.9g, of which saturates 0.3g; Cholesterol 0mg; Calcium 13mg; Fibre 0.9g; Sodium 29mg. **402** calories

Vegetable sauce with pasta: per portion Energy 440kcal/1839kJ; Protein 1.5g; Carbohydrate 6.5g, of which sugars 6.1g; Fat 4.3g, of which saturates 0.7g; Cholesterol 0mg; Calcium 15mg; Fibre 3.7g; Sodium 7mg. **440** calories

Pesto sauce with pasta: per portion Energy 529kcal/2203kJ; Protein 2.8g; Carbohydrate 0.7g, of which sugars 0.3g; Fat 16g, of which saturates 2.8g; Cholesterol 5mg; Calcium 73mg; Fibre 0.2g; Sodium 39mg. **529** calories

Nut cream sauce with pasta: per portion Energy 508kcal/2126kJ; Protein 4.8g; Carbohydrate 4.5g, of which sugars 0g; Fat 12.3g, of which saturates 1.4g; Cholesterol 0mg; Calcium 0mg; Fibre 3.7g; Sodium 0mg. **508** calories

Courgetti carbonara

In this pasta-free carbonara, courgettes are spiralized using a special machine, but you can just create ribbons with a peeler if you don't own a spiralizer.

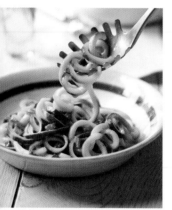

serves 4

115g/4oz pancetta or
   lean bacon, chopped
1 garlic clove, peeled
   and finely chopped
4 courgettes (zucchini)
2 eggs
4 egg yolks
50g/2oz/⅔ cup grated
   Parmesan cheese
ground black pepper,
   to taste

1 Stir-fry the pancetta in a large non-stick frying pan for 3–4 minutes, until crisp. Add the garlic and stir for 30 seconds. Transfer to kitchen paper.

2 Spiralize the courgettes, if you have a spiralizer, or shave them into ribbons using a vegetable peeler. Bring a pan of water to the boil, add the courgettes and cook for 2–3 minutes, until barely tender. Drain, reserving 75ml/5 tbsp of the water.

3 Beat together the eggs, yolks, Parmesan and pepper. Stir in the warm reserved cooking water.

4 Stir-fry the courgettes in the frying pan for 1 minute. Turn off the heat. Add the egg mixture, stirring until the sauce is thickened. Stir in the pancetta and serve immediately on warmed plates.

Per portion Energy 244kcal/1012kJ; Protein 18g; Carbohydrate 3.9g, of which sugars 3.5g; Fat 17.4g, of which saturates 6.7g; Cholesterol 247mg; Calcium 209mg; Fibre 2.5g; Sodium 505mg.

244
calories

Seven-flavour pasta

Ripe tomatoes are perfectly balanced by the seven flavours of garlic, olive oil, basil, parsley, oregano, onion and celery in this make-ahead summer dish.

serves 4

600g/1lb 5oz ripe tomatoes
1 garlic clove, peeled and crushed
45ml/3 tbsp olive oil
10 fresh basil leaves, torn into small shreds
30ml/2 tbsp chopped fresh parsley
5ml/1 tsp dried oregano
½ onion, peeled and very finely chopped
1 celery stick, very finely chopped
400g/14oz macaroni or other pasta shapes
salt and ground black pepper, to taste

1 Score the tomatoes with an 'X'. Plunge them into boiling water for 30 seconds, then refresh in cold water. Peel away the skins. Cut them in half and remove the seeds. Quarter and place in a colander set over a bowl and drain for 30 minutes.

2 Discard the juice (or save for use elsewhere) and put the tomatoes in a bowl. Mix in the garlic, olive oil, basil, parsley, oregano, onion and celery. Season and leave to stand overnight or for at least 2 hours.

3 When you are ready to serve, cook the pasta according to the pack instructions until al dente.

4 Drain the pasta and return it to the pan. Pour over the tomato sauce and stir together. Serve immediately. As the sauce is served cold, the dish will be lukewarm.

Per portion Energy 460kcal/1946kJ; Protein 14.3g; Carbohydrate 81.3g, of which sugars 9.7g; Fat 10.9g, of which saturates 1.5g; Cholesterol 0mg; Calcium 101mg; Fibre 8.2g; Sodium 31mg.

460
calories

Baked macaroni cheese

It is definitely worth knowing how to cook this classic dish. Once you've made the sauce for this you'll be able to make white sauces for all kinds of recipes, and home-made ones are much healthier than store-bought versions. Use brown breadcrumbs and wholemeal macaroni for added fibre.

serves 4
· · · · · · · · · ·

500ml/16fl oz/2 cups semi-skimmed (low-fat) milk
1 bay leaf
50g/2oz/4 tbsp unsalted butter
30ml/2 tbsp plain (all-purpose) flour
salt and ground black pepper, to taste
a pinch of nutmeg (optional)
175g/6oz/1½ cups freshly grated low-fat
  Cheddar cheese
40g/1¾oz/⅓ cup fresh brown or white
  breadcrumbs
450g/1lb white or wholemeal (whole-wheat)
  elbow macaroni

1 Put the milk in a small pan with the bay leaf. Heat gently, remove from the heat and strain into a jug or pitcher.

2 Melt the butter in a medium pan. Add the flour and whisk. Cook, whisking, for 2–3 minutes, then remove from the heat.

3 Gradually mix the milk into the butter and flour mixture. Return to the heat and bring to the boil, beating, until thickened. Remove the pan from the heat and season with salt and pepper, adding the nutmeg, if using.

4 Add all but 30ml/2 tbsp of the cheese and stir until melted. Transfer to a heatproof bowl. Cover with a layer of clear film or plastic wrap. Set aside.

5 Fill a large pan with water and bring to the boil. Preheat the oven to 200°C/400°F/Gas 6.

6 Grease an ovenproof dish and sprinkle with some of the breadcrumbs.

7 Add the macaroni to the pan of boiling water, and cook according to the packet instructions until it is just tender (al dente).

8 Drain the macaroni in a colander. Combine it with the sauce and transfer to the dish. Sprinkle the top with the remaining breadcrumbs and cheese. Bake for 20 minutes, until golden.

Per portion Energy 716kcal/3022kJ; Protein 33.9g; Carbohydrate 103.2g, of which sugars 10.3g; Fat 21.5g, of which saturates 12.5g; Cholesterol 54mg; Calcium 559mg; Fibre 5g; Sodium 511mg.

716 calories

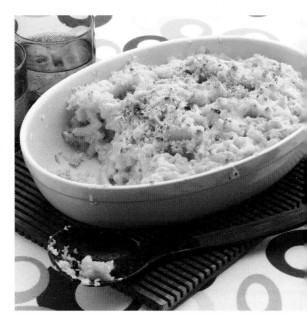

Spudtastic

Baked potatoes are easy to cook, and served with these toppings they're a real treat. The red bean chilli and the cheese and creamy corn toppings also make brilliant fillings for quesadillas (see page 94), and they can all be used in wraps. The stir-fried veg can be accompanied by noodles or rice, too.

each serves 4
. . . .

4 medium baking potatoes
a filling of your choice (see below)

for the stir-fried veg
30ml/2 tbsp sunflower oil
2 leeks, thinly sliced
2 carrots, peeled and cut into sticks
1 courgette (zucchini), thinly sliced
115g/4oz baby corn, halved
115g/4oz/1½ cups button (white) mushrooms, wiped clean and sliced
15ml/1 tbsp soy sauce
30ml/2 tbsp water
5ml/1 tsp sesame oil
sesame seeds, to garnish

for the red bean chilli
425g/15oz can red kidney beans, drained
200g/7oz/scant 1 cup low-fat cottage cheese
30ml/2 tbsp mild chilli sauce, plus extra (optional)
5ml/1 tsp ground cumin

for the cheese and creamy corn
425g/15oz canned corn, drained
50g/2oz/½ cup grated low-fat Cheddar cheese
5ml/1 tsp mixed dried herbs
fresh parsley sprigs, to garnish

1 Preheat the oven to 200°C/400°F/Gas 6. Prick the potatoes all over and place on a baking sheet and cook for 45–60 minutes, until soft and cooked through. Alternatively, microwave the potatoes (see cook's tip).

2 Remove the cooked potatoes from the oven or microwave and leave them on a plate to cool down slightly for a few minutes, so they are safe to handle. Meanwhile, make the chosen topping.

3 To make the **stir-fried veg**, heat the oil in a wok or large frying pan over a high heat.

4 Add the leeks, carrots, courgette and baby corn to the wok or pan and stir-fry together for about 2 minutes, then add the mushrooms and stir-fry for a further 1 minute.

5 Mix together the soy sauce, water and sesame oil in a small bowl. Pour the mixture over the vegetables in the wok or frying pan. Heat until the sauce is just bubbling, then scatter over the sesame seeds.

6 To make the **red bean chilli**, heat the drained red kidney beans in a small pan for 5 minutes or in a microwave for about 3 minutes, until they are hot.

7 Stir in the cottage cheese, chilli sauce and cumin. Heat for 1 minute.

8 To make the **cheese and creamy corn** filling, heat the corn in a small pan with the cheese and herbs for about 5 minutes, until hot. Blitz until creamy with a hand-held blender.

9 Place the potatoes on a chopping board and cut them open in a cross shape with a knife. Push up the flesh.

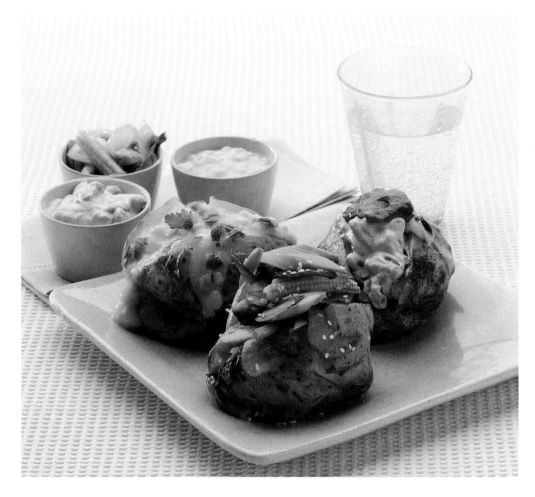

10 Fill with stir-fried veg; spoon on the red bean chilli and top with more chilli sauce, if you like things spicy; or spoon on the cheese and creamy corn filling and garnish with fresh parsley sprigs.

cook's tip

• To microwave the potatoes, cook them on a microwave-safe plate for 10 minutes. Turn them over and cook for a further 10 minutes, or until done. If you are microwaving just 1 potato, cook for 5 minutes, turn, and cook for 5 minutes more.

Stir-fried veg: per portion Energy 266kcal/1120kJ; Protein 7.3g; Carbohydrate 39.5g, of which sugars 8.8g; Fat 9.8g, of which saturates 1.5g; Cholesterol 66mg; Calcium 58mg; Fibre 8g; Sodium 630mg.

266 calories

Red bean chilli: per portion Energy 261kcal/1106kJ; Protein 15.6g; Carbohydrate 48.5g, of which sugars 8.3g; Fat 2.1g, of which saturates 0.8g; Cholesterol 69mg; Calcium 142mg; Fibre 9g; Sodium 663mg.

261 calories

Cheese and creamy corn: per portion Energy 258kcal/1095kJ; Protein 10.7g; Carbohydrate 47.3g, of which sugars 4.5g; Fat 4.2g, of which saturates 1.6g; Cholesterol 71mg; Calcium 133mg; Fibre 4.9g; Sodium 109mg.

258 calories

Roasted vegetables

Roasting the vegetables brings out their flavour, and the addition of thyme and a sprinkling of cumin seeds removes the need for added salt.

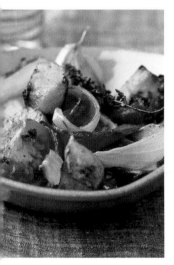

serves 4

3 courgettes (zucchini)
1 large fennel bulb
1 onion, peeled
2 red (bell) peppers
450g/1lb butternut squash
6 garlic cloves
60ml/4 tbsp olive oil
juice of ½ lemon
a pinch of cumin seeds
ground black pepper, to taste
4 sprigs fresh thyme
4 medium tomatoes

1 Preheat the oven to 220°C/425°F/Gas 7. Cut all the vegetables into large bitesize pieces. Smash the garlic with the flat of a knife, but leave the skins on.

2 Choose a roasting pan large enough to fit all the vegetables (except the tomatoes) in one layer. Mix together the oil and lemon juice. Pour over the vegetables and toss well. Sprinkle with the cumin seeds and pepper and tuck in the thyme sprigs. Roast for 20 minutes.

3 Add the tomatoes and gently stir. Cook for a further 15 minutes, or until the vegetables are tender and slightly charred around the edges.

Per portion Energy 213Kcal/883kJ; Protein 5.7g; Carbohydrate 20.3g, of which sugars 17.5g; Fat 12.6g, of which saturates 2g; Cholesterol 0mg; Calcium 109mg; Fibre 7.3g; Sodium 24mg.

213 calories

Courgette and potato bake

This dish is great served with wholemeal bread and a crisp green salad. It is easy to make, satisfying and looks good when brought to the table.

serves 6

675g/1½lb courgettes (zucchini), cut into rounds
450g/1lb potatoes, peeled and cut into chunks
1 onion, peeled and roughly chopped
3 garlic cloves, peeled and chopped
1 large red (bell) pepper, seeded and chopped
400g/14oz can chopped tomatoes
60ml/4 tbsp olive oil
250ml/8fl oz/1 cup hot water
5ml/1 tsp dried oregano
salt and ground black pepper, to taste
45ml/3 tbsp chopped fresh flat leaf parsley

1 Preheat the oven to 190°C/375°F/Gas 5.

2 Put the courgettes, potatoes, onion, garlic, pepper and tomatoes in a baking dish and mix well to combine, then stir in the olive oil, hot water and dried oregano.

3 Spread the mixture evenly, then season to taste with salt and pepper. Bake for 30 minutes.

4 Stir in the parsley and a little more water if necessary, and cook for 1 hour, increasing the temperature to 200°C/400°F/Gas 6 for the final 10–15 minutes, so that the potatoes brown.

5 Remove from the oven and cool for 5 minutes before serving garnished with parsley.

Per portion Energy 171kcal/715kJ; Protein 4.7g; Carbohydrate 20.4g, of which sugars 8g; Fat 8.4g, of which saturates 1.3g; Cholesterol 25mg; Calcium 67mg; Fibre 4.2g; Sodium 38mg.

171 calories

Potato and tomato bake

The humble potato is sliced and layered with red onion, tomato and breadcrumbs to make this easy, comforting dish. It's ideal for lunch, served with a salad.

serves 4–6

4 large potatoes, peeled
60ml/4 tbsp olive oil, plus extra for greasing
25ml/1½ tbsp dried oregano
60ml/4 tbsp fresh white breadcrumbs
salt and ground black pepper, to taste
3 very large, ripe tomatoes, sliced
3 red onions, peeled and thinly sliced into rings
salad, to serve

1 Boil the potatoes for 4 minutes, then drain and slice into thin discs.

2 Grease a shallow ovenproof dish (large enough to hold all the vegetables) with olive oil.

3 Arrange a layer of potatoes on the bottom of the dish. Sprinkle with oregano, a little olive oil and a few pinches of breadcrumbs, then season.

4 Cover with a layer of tomatoes and a layer of onions, topped with seasoning, oil and breadcrumbs. Repeat until all the vegetables have been used up, finishing with a coating of breadcrumbs.

5 Leave the dish to stand while you preheat the oven to 180°C/350°F/Gas 4.

6 Bake for 30 minutes, or until the top is browned and crisp. Serve warm with salad.

Per portion Energy 265kcal/1115kJ; Protein 5.7g; Carbohydrate 43.9g, of which sugars 8.2g; Fat 8.7g, of which saturates 1.4g; Cholesterol 55mg; Calcium 103mg; Fibre 4.6g; Sodium 102mg.

265 calories

Baked eggs with tomatoes

This really is a delightfully simple dish, and it comes from Italy. It's good served with plenty of wholemeal bread and a green salad.

serves 4

500g/1¼lb/2½ cups canned chopped tomatoes
30ml/2 tbsp water
salt and ground black pepper, to taste
15ml/1 tbsp extra virgin olive oil
1 garlic clove, peeled and finely chopped
8 eggs
chopped parsley, to garnish
salad, to serve

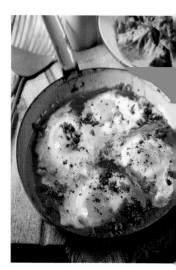

1 Put the tomatoes into a pan with the water and a pinch of salt. Cover and simmer gently for 30 minutes, stirring occasionally.

2 Preheat the oven to 200°C/400°F/Gas 6. Push the tomato sauce through a strainer.

3 Pour the oil into an ovenproof frying pan, add the garlic and fry gently for 2–3 minutes. Pour over the tomato sauce, break the eggs on top of the sauce and sprinkle with pepper.

4 Bake in the oven for 5 minutes, until the eggs are set. Garnish with parsley and serve with a salad.

Per portion Energy 243kcal/1008kJ; Protein 13.4g; Carbohydrate 3.9g, of which sugars 3.9g; Fat 19.7g, of which saturates 4.4g; Cholesterol 381mg; Calcium 66mg; Fibre 1.3g; Sodium 151mg.

243 calories

Tomato and lentil dhal

Delicious, nutritious and very versatile, dhal is a mainstay of Indian cuisine and deserves to appear more frequently on supper tables across the world. The addition of tomatoes in this one makes it more palatable for children, and you can adjust the spices to suit your family. Serve as an accompaniment or as a main with wholemeal bread.

serves 4

30ml/2 tbsp vegetable oil
1 large onion, peeled and finely chopped
3 garlic cloves, peeled and chopped
1 carrot, peeled and diced
10ml/2 tsp cumin seeds
10ml/2 tsp mustard seeds
2.5cm/1in fresh root ginger, grated
10ml/2 tsp ground turmeric
5ml/1 tsp mild chilli powder
5ml/1 tsp garam masala
225g/8oz/1 cup split red lentils
800ml/1½ pints/3¼ cups low-salt stock or water
5 tomatoes, peeled, seeded and chopped
ground black pepper, to taste
juice of 2 limes
60ml/4 tbsp chopped fresh coriander (cilantro)
25g/1oz/¼ cup flaked (sliced) almonds

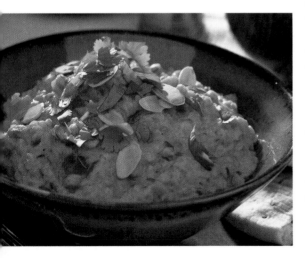

1 Heat the oil in a heavy pan. Sauté the onion over a medium heat for about 10 minutes, until softened, stirring occasionally.

2 Add the garlic, carrot, cumin and mustard seeds, and ginger. Cook for 10 minutes, stirring, until the seeds pop and the carrot softens slightly.

3 Stir in the ground turmeric, chilli powder and garam masala and cook the mixture on a low heat for 1 minute or until the flavours begin to mingle, stirring continuously to prevent the spices from burning.

4 Add the lentils, stock or water and seeded and chopped tomatoes, and season to taste with pepper.

5 Bring to the boil, then reduce the heat and simmer, covered, for about 45 minutes, stirring occasionally to prevent the mixture from sticking to the bottom of the pan.

6 Stir in the lime juice and 45ml/3 tbsp of the chopped fresh coriander. Cook for a further 15 minutes, until the lentils are tender.

7 Toast the almonds in a hot pan for 3–4 minutes, shaking the pan to prevent them from burning.

8 Sprinkle the dhal with the remaining coriander and the flaked almonds and serve immediately.

Per portion Energy 335kcal/1404kJ; Protein 18.7g; Carbohydrate 44.3g, of which sugars 10.5g; Fat 13g, of which saturates 1.5g; Cholesterol 0mg; Calcium 189mg; Fibre 7.7g; Sodium 57mg.

335 calories

Giant baked beans

Kids who like canned baked beans will love these home-made giant ones! Serve as a main dish with a green vegetable, or in smaller portions as an accompaniment.

serves 4

45ml/3 tbsp olive oil
2 onions, peeled and finely chopped
1 celery stick, thinly sliced
2 carrots, peeled and diced
3 garlic cloves, peeled and thinly sliced
5ml/1 tsp each dried oregano and thyme
400g/14oz can chopped tomatoes
30ml/2 tbsp tomato purée (paste) diluted in
    300ml/½ pint/1¼ cups hot water
400g/14oz/1¾ canned large white
    beans, drained
30ml/2 tbsp apple juice
45ml/3 tbsp finely chopped flat leaf parsley
ground black pepper, to taste

1 Preheat the oven to 180°C/350°F/Gas 4. Heat the oil in a pan, add the onions and sauté for 10 minutes. Add the celery, carrots, garlic and herbs and stir until the garlic becomes aromatic.

2 Stir in the tomatoes, cover and cook for 10 minutes. Pour in the tomato purée, then add the beans, apple juice, half the parsley and pepper.

3 Transfer the bean mixture into a large baking dish and bake for 30 minutes, checking the beans once or twice and adding more hot water if they look dry; they should just be moist. Stir in the remaining parsley and serve.

Per portion Energy 205kcal/860kJ; Protein 7.3g; Carbohydrate 24.8g, of which sugars 12.6g; Fat 9.3g, of which saturates 1.4g; Cholesterol 0mg; Calcium 112mg; Fibre 8.8g; Sodium 391mg.

205 calories

Braised beans and lentils

High in soluble fibre and protein, this braised dish packs a real nutritional punch. Leave off the onion and dill topping if you prefer.

serves 4

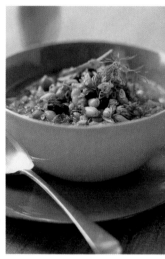

150g/5oz/¾ cup dried
    mixed beans,
    soaked overnight
75g/3oz/⅔ cup brown or
    green lentils
15ml/1 tbsp olive oil
1 onion, finely chopped
2 garlic cloves, crushed
6 sage leaves, chopped
juice of 1 lemon
ground black pepper
3 spring onions (scallions),
    thinly sliced
60ml/4 tbsp chopped dill

1 Drain the beans and place in a large pan. Cover with cold water, bring to the boil, and cook for 1 hour. Add the lentils and cook for 30 minutes.

2 Drain, reserving the cooking liquid. Return the beans and lentils to the pan.

3 Heat the oil in a frying pan and fry the onion until golden. Add the garlic and sage, cook for 30 seconds, then add to the beans. Stir in the reserved liquid and simmer for 15 minutes.

4 Stir in the lemon juice and season to taste with pepper. Serve topped with spring onions and dill.

Per portion Energy 223Kcal/945kJ; Protein 14.4g; Carbohydrate 34.9g, of which sugars 5.4g; Fat 3.9g, of which saturates 0.6g; Cholesterol 0mg; Calcium 95mg; Fibre 7.9g; Sodium 13mg.

223 calories

Fast fishes

These little fishes will appeal to even the fussiest younger diner. Use a sustainable type of white fish instead of salmon fillet, if you like, although oily fish is healthiest.

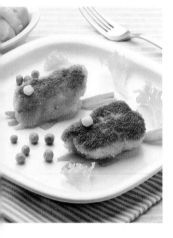

serves 2

6 new potatoes
30ml/2 tbsp frozen peas
4 frozen corn kernels
2 salmon fillets, each
    75g/3oz, skinned
1 carrot, peeled
1 egg
115ml/4oz/2 cups fresh
    breadcrumbs
20ml/4 tsp sesame
    seeds
20ml/4 tsp vegetable oil

1 Put the potatoes in a pan of boiling water and cook for 10–15 minutes, until soft. Add the peas and corn for the last 3 minutes, then drain.

2 Meanwhile, cut the fish into four pieces. Cut the carrot into long thin slices, then cut out fin and tail shapes and tiny triangles for mouth parts.

3 Put the egg in a dish and whisk it. Mix the breadcrumbs and sesame seeds on a plate. Dip the fish in egg then in the breadcrumbs, to coat.

4 Fry the fish in the oil for 3–4 minutes per side, until golden brown all over. Put the fish on plates, position the carrot pieces, and use the corn as eyes and peas as bubbles. Serve with the potatoes.

Per portion Energy 582kcal/2441kJ; Protein 29.3g; Carbohydrate 61.4g, of which sugars5.7g; Fat 26g, of which saturates 4.4g; Cholesterol 159mg; Calcium 189mg; Fibre 5.9g; Sodium 534mg.

582 calories

Tuna and corn fishcakes

This simple recipe is a lovely way to use up leftover mashed potatoes. If you like, try making fish- or star-shaped cakes using cookie cutters.

serves 4

350g/12oz floury potatoes, peeled and cubed
200g/7oz can tuna fish, drained
115g/4oz/¾ cup canned or frozen corn
30ml/2 tbsp chopped fresh parsley
salt and ground black pepper, to taste
225g/8oz/4 cups fresh wholemeal (whole-wheat)
    breadcrumbs
30ml/2 tbsp vegetable oil
grilled (broiled) tomatoes and salad, to serve

1 Put the potatoes in a large pan and cover with cold water. Bring to the boil and boil for 10–15 minutes or until tender.

2 Drain the potatoes, then return to the pan. Mash until smooth and set aside to cool.

3 Place the mashed potatoes in a bowl and stir in the tuna, corn and parsley. Season to taste and combine thoroughly. Divide the mixture into eight portions. Form these into patty shapes with damp hands (to prevent the mixture sticking).

4 Spread out the breadcrumbs on a plate. Press the fishcakes into the breadcrumbs to coat evenly.

5 Heat the oil in a frying pan, add the cakes and cook for 2 minutes on each side, until golden brown. Serve with grilled tomatoes and salad.

Per portion Energy 255kcal/1081kJ; Protein 13.2g; Carbohydrate 41.7g, of which sugars 2.1g; Fat 5.1g, of which saturates 0.6g; Cholesterol 35mg; Calcium 55mg; Fibre 2.3g; Sodium 390mg.

255 calories

Roasted fish

Oily fish such as salmon, mackerel and sardines are good sources of Omega 3 fats. The tomato sauce in this dish will make the fish more appealing for children.

serves 4

350g/12oz ripe tomatoes
30ml/2 tbsp olive oil
2 strips of pared orange rind
1 fresh thyme sprig
6 fresh basil leaves
450g/1lb oily fish fillet, such as salmon, skin descaled
steamed French (green) beans, to serve

1 Preheat the oven to 230°C/450°F/Gas 8. Using a small, sharp knife, roughly chop the tomatoes, leaving their skins on, and set aside.

2 Heat 15ml/1 tbsp of the oil in a heavy pan, add the tomatoes, orange rind, thyme and basil, and simmer for 5 minutes, until the tomatoes are soft and juicy. Press through a fine sieve or strainer, pour the smooth sauce into a pan and heat gently.

3 Cut the fish into four even-size pieces. Brush a griddle with the remaining oil, then cook the fish skin-side down for 5 minutes, until it is almost cooked all the way through.

4 Flip over the fish and cook for 1–2 minutes, until cooked through.

5 Serve on top of the steamed French beans with the fresh tomato sauce.

Per portion Energy 267kcal/1111kJ; Protein 23.4g; Carbohydrate 2.7g, of which sugars 2.7g; Fat 18.1g, of which saturates 3g; Cholesterol 56mg; Calcium 30mg; Fibre 1.2g; Sodium 59mg.

267 calories

Fish kebabs

These succulent kebabs make a healthy alternative to burgers or sausages for a summer barbecue. You can swap the fish for cubed chicken breast fillets.

serves 4

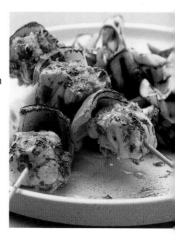

3 garlic cloves, chopped
2.5ml/½ tsp paprika
2.5ml/½ tsp ground cumin
2.5ml/½ tsp salt
60ml/4 tbsp olive oil
30ml/2 tbsp lemon juice
30ml/2 tbsp chopped fresh parsley
450g/1lb firm white fish fillet, cut into cubes
2 green (bell) peppers, cut into pieces

1 Put the garlic, paprika, cumin, salt, oil, lemon juice and parsley in a large bowl and mix together. Add the fish and toss to coat completely.

2 Cover with clear film or plastic wrap and leave to marinate for at least 1 hour.

3 Prepare a barbecue (it is ready when the coals have turned white and grey) or preheat a griddle on the stove.

4 Thread the fish cubes and pepper pieces alternately on to wooden skewers (soaked in water for 30 minutes first) or metal skewers. Cook for 2–3 minutes on each side, or until the fish is lightly browned.

Per portion Energy 260kcal/1089kJ; Protein 28.2g; Carbohydrate 9.5g, of which sugars 9g; Fat 12.4g, of which saturates 1.9g; Cholesterol 24mg; Calcium 45mg; Fibre 2.8g; Sodium 40mg.

260 calories

Fish and bean stew

Everything is cooked in one pot in this divine dish, which combines fresh white fish with sweet tomatoes and soft beans. You can use whichever beans you happen to have in the storecupboard or pantry, and a sustainable type of fish.

serves 4

1 red (bell) pepper
45ml/3 tbsp olive oil
1 onion, peeled and sliced
2 garlic cloves, peeled and chopped
10ml/2 tsp paprika
400g/14oz can haricot (navy) beans,
    drained and rinsed
about 600ml/1 pint/2½ cups low-salt fish stock
6 tomatoes, quartered
350g/12oz skinned white fish fillet,
    cut into chunks
salt and ground black pepper, to taste
45ml/3 tbsp chopped fresh coriander (cilantro),
    plus a few sprigs to garnish
wholemeal (whole-wheat) bread and salad, to serve

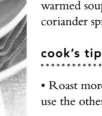

1 Preheat the grill (broiler) and line the pan with foil. Halve the red pepper and scoop out the seeds. Place the halves, cut side down, in the pan and cook under a hot grill for 10–15 minutes, until the skin is charred. Alternatively, you can hold the pepper with tongs and insert it directly into a gas flame, turning it until the skin blisters and blackens slightly all over.

2 Put the pepper into a plastic bag, seal it and leave it for 10 minutes to steam. Remove from the bag, peel off the skin and discard. Chop the pepper into large pieces.

3 Heat the oil in a pan, then add the onion. Fry for 2 minutes, then add the garlic. Cover and cook for 10 minutes, until the onion is soft.

4 Stir in the paprika and beans and add enough stock to cover. Bring to the boil and simmer, uncovered, for 15 minutes. Stir in the red pepper and tomato. Add the fish and cover with the sauce.

5 Cover and simmer for 5 minutes, then season to taste. Stir in the chopped coriander. Serve in warmed soup plates or bowls, garnished with the coriander sprigs. Serve with bread and salad.

cook's tip

• Roast more than 1 (bell) pepper at a time, and use the others in salads or other dishes.

Per portion Energy 285kcal/1192kJ; Protein 23.4g; Carbohydrate 24.9g, of which sugars 11.1g; Fat 10.8g, of which saturates 1.7g; Cholesterol 40mg; Calcium 87mg; Fibre 9.3g; Sodium 359mg.

285 calories

Easy as fish pie

This creamy mixture of fish and corn topped with potato, cabbage and cheese is easy to make, warming and filling – perfect for a winter's day. This dish freezes very well, so cook twice the quantity and freeze half for another time.

serves 4
. . . .

4 potatoes, peeled and chopped
50g/2oz green cabbage
250g/8oz fish pie mixture
300ml/½ pint/1¼ cups semi-skimmed (low-fat) milk
30ml/2 tbsp unsalted butter
30ml/2 tbsp plain (all-purpose) flour
75g/3oz/6 tbsp frozen corn
50g/2oz/½ cup low-fat Cheddar cheese, grated
10ml/2 tsp sesame seeds
cooked carrot sticks and mangetouts (snow peas), to serve

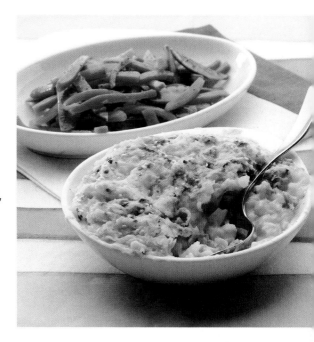

1 Three-quarters fill a large pan with water and bring to the boil. Add the chopped potato and cook for 10 minutes. Add the cabbage and cook for 5 minutes more, until the potatoes are tender.

2 Drain the potatoes and cabbage in a colander. Return to the pan and cover with a lid.

3 Meanwhile, place the fish pie mixture and all but 45ml/3 tbsp of the milk in another large pan. Bring to the boil, then cover, reduce the heat and simmer very gently for 8–10 minutes, until the fish flakes easily when pressed with the tip of a table knife.

4 Drain the fish over a large bowl, reserving the milk. Wash the pan.

5 Melt the butter in the clean pan. Stir in the flour and cook, stirring, for 1–2 minutes. Stir in the reserved milk (from step 4). Return to the heat and bring to the boil, stirring until thickened.

6 Preheat the grill (broiler) to medium-hot. Add the fish and corn to the sauce with half the cheese. Spoon into four small dishes or one large one.

7 Mash the cooked potato and cabbage with the remaining fresh milk. Stir in half the remaining cheese. Spoon the mixture over the fish and sprinkle with sesame seeds and the remaining cheese.

8 Place under the hot grill and cook until the topping is browned. Serve with the vegetables.

Per portion Energy 341kcal/1433kJ; Protein 21.3g; Carbohydrate 33.4g, of which sugars 6.3g; Fat 14.5g, of which saturates 8g; Cholesterol 103mg; Calcium 224mg; Fibre 3.1g; Sodium 226mg.

341
calories

Pan-fried chicken with pesto

This dish is a firm family favourite and makes a very nutritious meal. Half a chicken breast fillet will be enough for most younger children.

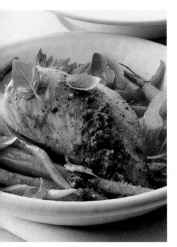

serves 4–6
....

15ml/1 tbsp olive oil
4 skinless chicken
    breast fillets
roasted baby vegetables

For the pesto
90ml/6 tbsp olive oil
50g/2oz/½ cup pine nuts
50g/2oz/1 cup basil
15g/½oz/¼ cup parsley
2 garlic cloves, crushed
ground black pepper,
    to taste

1 Heat the 15ml/1 tbsp oil in a frying pan. Add the chicken and cook gently for 15–20 minutes, turning often, until lightly browned and cooked.

2 Meanwhile, make the pesto. Place the oil, pine nuts, basil, parsley, garlic and pepper in a blender or food processor and process until smooth.

3 Remove the chicken from the pan, cover and keep hot. Reduce the heat slightly, then add the pesto to the pan and cook gently, stirring, for a few minutes until the pesto has warmed through.

4 Pour the warm pesto over the chicken and serve with roasted vegetables.

Per portion Energy 265kcal/1103kJ; Protein 21.5g; Carbohydrate 0.8g, of which sugars 0.4g; Fat 19.6g, of which saturates 2.5g; Cholesterol 58mg; Calcium 31mg; Fibre 0.4g; Sodium 52mg.

265
calories

Griddled chicken with salsa

This aromatic dish is a great way to enjoy the flavour, colour and health benefits of good-quality fresh ingredients. For best results, marinate the chicken overnight.

serves 3–4
....

3 skinless chicken breast fillets
30ml/2 tbsp fresh lemon juice
30ml/2 tbsp olive oil
10ml/2 tsp ground cumin
10ml/2 tsp dried oregano
15ml/1 tbsp ground black pepper, to taste

For the salsa
450g/1lb plum tomatoes, seeded and chopped
3 spring onions (scallions), chopped
30ml/2 tbsp chopped fresh coriander (cilantro)
15ml/1 tbsp chopped fresh parsley
45ml/3 tbsp olive oil
30ml/2 tbsp fresh lemon juice

1 With a rolling pin, pound the chicken between two sheets of clear film or plastic wrap until thin. Halve any fillets intended for younger children.

2 In a shallow dish, combine the lemon juice, oil, cumin, oregano and pepper. Add the chicken, cover and leave to marinate for at least 2 hours.

3 To make the salsa, mix together all the ingredients.

4 Remove the chicken from the marinade. Heat a griddle pan. Cook the chicken for 4 minutes on each side, or until browned all over and cooked through. Serve with the tomato salsa.

Per portion Energy 225kcal/941kJ; Protein 23.9g; Carbohydrate 4.2g, of which sugars 4.2g; Fat 12.6g, of which saturates 2g; Cholesterol 66mg; Calcium 46mg; Fibre 2.7g; Sodium 72mg.

225
calories

Chicken casserole with vegetables

A casserole of wonderfully tender slow-cooked chicken, vegetables and zesty lemon, finished with fragrant herbs, this is the sort of dish that is ideally suited to family life, since the flavour improves if the dish is made in advance and stored in the refrigerator for a day or two before being reheated and served.

serves 6

30ml/2 tbsp vegetable oil
1 large chicken, cut into portions
1 onion, peeled and chopped
40g/1½oz/⅓ cup plain (all-purpose) flour
salt and ground black pepper
about 1.2 litres/2 pints/5 cups chicken or
    vegetable stock
2 carrots, peeled and cut into large chunks
1 garlic clove, peeled
bunch of fresh parsley
1 fresh thyme sprig
1 fresh marjoram sprig
grated rind and juice of 1 lemon
½ cauliflower, broken into florets
115g/4oz/1 cup peas
boiled or roasted new potatoes, to serve

1 Heat the oil in a large flameproof casserole dish or stockpot. Brown the chicken pieces all over, removing them from the pan when they are browned and setting them aside in a bowl.

2 Add the onion to the pot and cook, stirring often, for 5 minutes, until softened. Stir in the flour and cook, stirring constantly, until the mixture is lightly browned. Season, then gradually blend in the stock. Cook, stirring, for 1 minute, then bring to the boil and cook, stirring, until it is smooth.

3 Add the carrots and the garlic clove. Tie the parsley, thyme and marjoram together and add to the pan with the lemon rind and half the juice. Add the chicken with any juices from the bowl.

4 Slowly bring to the boil, then reduce the heat so that it simmers gently – check that all the chicken portions are covered with liquid; rearrange the portions or add a little extra stock if necessary.

5 Cover and simmer for about 1 hour, until everything is tender. Add the cauliflower and peas halfway through the cooking, distributing them evenly over the top. Bring the liquid back to a simmer before continuing to time the cooking.

6 To boost the tanginess, add the remaining lemon juice before serving with potatoes.

Per portion Energy 441kcal/1832kJ; Protein 35.5g;
Carbohydrate 13.6g, of which sugars 5.7g; Fat
27.4g, of which saturates 6.9g; Cholesterol 165mg;
Calcium 51mg; Fibre 4.2g; Sodium 398mg.

441
calories

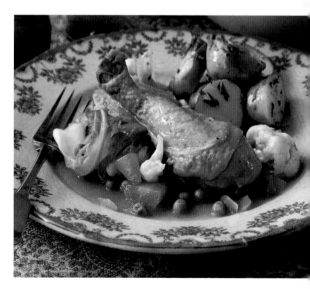

Turkey and corn stew

Turkey tends to be leaner than chicken and has an excellent fat profile, so it is a great alternative. The sweetness of the corn makes this an appealing dish for children.

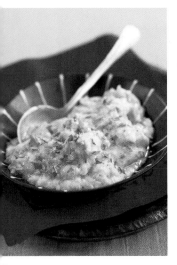

serves 4

175g/6oz/1 cup corn
30ml/2 tbsp oil
450g/1lb skinless turkey
    breast fillet, cut into
    2cm/¾in pieces
1 onion, finely chopped
2 garlic cloves, crushed
500ml/17fl oz/generous
    2 cups low-salt stock
ground black pepper
chopped parsley,
    to garnish
cooked brown rice,
    to serve

1 Blend the corn to a smooth purée in a food processor. Set aside.

2 Heat the oil in a large pan and fry the turkey over a high heat for 8–10 minutes, until golden.

3 Stir in the onion and garlic, reduce the heat slightly and cook for about 20 minutes, stirring frequently, until the onion is caramelized.

4 Pour in the stock. Bring to the boil and simmer for 20 minutes. Add the pepper and puréed corn and simmer for a further 15 minutes, until thick. Garnish with parsley and serve with brown rice.

Per portion Energy 232kcal/971kJ; Protein 29.5g; Carbohydrate 11.6g, of which sugars 3.1g; Fat 7.8g, of which saturates 1.2g; Cholesterol 64mg; Calcium 15mg; Fibre 1.6g; Sodium 58mg.

232
calories

Tantalizing turkey burgers

These delicious fresh-tasting burgers are a good midweek supper served in buns with salad. They are a much healthier alternative to traditional beef burgers.

serves 6

1 small red onion
450g/1lb minced (ground) turkey
15ml/1 tbsp fresh thyme leaves
30ml/2 tbsp olive oil
salt and ground black pepper, to taste
6 burger buns, lightly toasted
green salad

1 Peel and finely chop the onion. Put it in a mixing bowl with the turkey.

2 Add the thyme leaves and 15ml/1 tbsp of the oil and season to taste with salt and ground black pepper. Cover and chill for up to 4 hours.

3 Divide the mixture into six equal portions and shape into round patties using damp hands. If the mixture starts to stick, dampen your hands again.

4 Preheat a griddle pan. Brush the patties with half of the remaining oil. Place the patties on the griddle pan and cook for 10–12 minutes.

5 Turn the patties over, brush with more oil, and cook for 10–12 minutes on the second side, or until cooked right through.

6 Slice the burger buns in half, insert a burger into each and top with some green salad.

Per portion Energy 327kcal/1382kJ; Protein 26.3g; Carbohydrate 42.9g, of which sugars 2.6g; Fat 6.8g, of which saturates 1.5g; Cholesterol 43mg; Calcium 132mg; Fibre 1.9g; Sodium 506mg.

327
calories

Bashed turkey with lime

Pounding lean turkey breasts with a mallet tenderizes the meat and also makes it cook really quickly. Marinating the meat in lime juice for an hour helps give it flavour, reducing the need for any salt, but if you are short of time you can just marinate it for 10 minutes while you make a salad and set the table.

serves 4

450g/1lb thin turkey steaks
10ml/2 tsp dried oregano
3 ripe limes, 2 juiced, 1 sliced into wedges
  (to serve)
45ml/3 tbsp extra virgin olive oil
salt and ground black pepper, to taste
1 garlic clove, peeled and finely chopped
tomato and basil salad, to serve

1 Place the turkey steaks between two sheets of clear film or plastic wrap and beat them with a meat mallet or rolling pin until they are as thin as possible.

2 Spread the turkey slices out in a shallow dish and sprinkle with the oregano. Drizzle with the lime juice and 15ml/1 tbsp olive oil and season with salt and pepper. Cover and leave to marinate at room temperature for about 1 hour.

3 Lift out the turkey slices and pat them dry with kitchen paper.

4 Pour the remaining olive oil into a frying pan. Add the garlic and heat over a high heat. When it sizzles, add as many of the turkey slices as the pan will hold in a single layer.

5 Fry the turkey slices for 1–2 minutes on each side, until just cooked through.

6 Transfer the turkey to heated plates and keep it hot while you cook the remaining slices.

7 Divide the juices remaining in the pan among the turkey slices, spooning them over the top. Garnish with the lime wedges and serve with a tomato and basil salad.

variations

• Orange or lemon juice could be used in place of lime, if you prefer.
• Instead of turkey steaks, try escalopes (US scallops) of chicken or veal, or thin slices of monkfish.

Per portion Energy 200kcal/837kJ; Protein 27.7g; Carbohydrate 1.3g, of which sugars 0g; Fat 9.4g, of which saturates 1.6g; Cholesterol 64mg; Calcium 44mg; Fibre 0g; Sodium 57mg.

200 calories

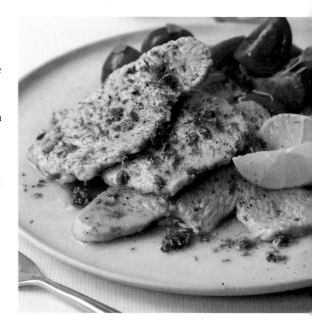

Skinny meatballs in tomato sauce

In this delicious dish, minced turkey is shaped into small balls and simmered in a richly flavoured tomato sauce, then served with rice. This recipe is very easy to double up, and freezes beautifully if you want to get ahead.

serves 4
. . . .

3 slices of wholemeal (whole-wheat) bread
30ml/2 tbsp semi-skimmed milk
1 garlic clove, crushed
2.5ml/½ tsp caraway seeds
225g/8oz minced (ground) turkey
salt and ground black pepper, to taste
1 egg white
350ml/12fl oz/1½ cups near-boiling low-salt stock
400g/14oz can chopped tomatoes
15ml/1 tbsp tomato purée (paste)
basmati rice and assorted steamed vegetables,
   to serve

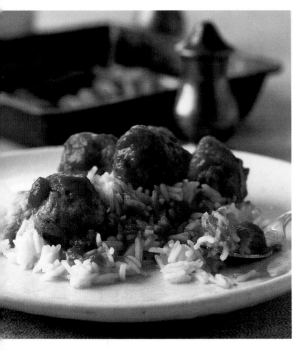

1 Using a serrated knife, remove the crusts from the bread and cut it into cubes. Place the bread in a mixing bowl and sprinkle with the milk, then leave to soak for about 5 minutes.

2 Add the garlic, caraway seeds, minced turkey and salt and pepper to the bread and mix together well.

3 Whisk the egg white until stiff, then fold it into the turkey mixture. Cover and chill in the refrigerator for 30 minutes.

4 Preheat the oven to 190°C/375°F/Gas 5. Pour the stock into a large ovenproof dish. Add the tomatoes and tomato purée, cover with a lid and cook for 30 minutes.

5 Meanwhile, shape the turkey mixture into 16 small balls. Drop them into the tomato sauce.

6 Cook for a further 30 minutes, or until the turkey balls are cooked. Serve immediately with some rice and steamed vegetables.

variations
. . . .

• You could make these meatballs using any type of lean minced (ground) meat, including chicken, pork, beef and lamb.
• Try adding some chopped courgette (zucchini) or (bell) pepper to the sauce in step 5.

Per portion Energy 140kcal/592kJ; Protein 18.1g; Carbohydrate 14.2g, of which sugars 4.4g; Fat 1.6g, of which saturates 0.5g; Cholesterol 33mg; Calcium 48mg; Fibre 2.7g; Sodium 205mg.

140
calories

Beef and mushroom burgers

Bulking out burgers with breadcrumbs and mushrooms reduces their fat and calorie content considerably.

serves 4

1 small onion, peeled and chopped
150g/5oz/2 cups mushrooms
450g/1lb very lean minced (ground) beef
50g/2oz/1 cup fresh wholemeal (whole-wheat) breadcrumbs
5ml/1 tsp dried mixed herbs
15ml/1 tbsp tomato purée (paste)
salt and ground black pepper, to taste
4 wholemeal (whole-wheat) burger buns or pitta breads
sliced gherkins and salad leaves

1 Place the onion and mushrooms in a food processor and process until finely chopped, or do it by hand.

2 Add the minced beef, fresh breadcrumbs, herbs, tomato purée and seasoning. Process for a few seconds, until the mixture binds together but still has some texture.

3 Divide the mixture into four, then press each portion into burgers using dampened hands.

4 Cook the burgers in a large non-stick frying pan or under a hot grill (broiler) for 12–15 minutes, turning once, until evenly cooked.

5 Serve in burger buns or pitta bread (lightly toasted, if you like) with gherkins and salad leaves.

Per portion Energy 265kcal/1110kJ; Protein 27.6g; Carbohydrate 13.8g, of which sugars 3g; Fat 11.4g, of which saturates 4.8g; Cholesterol 63mg; Calcium 61mg; Fibre 1.8g; Sodium 209mg.

265 calories

Thai pork patties

These zesty patties are a bit different from the usual burger and are much healthier and more flavoursome.

serves 4

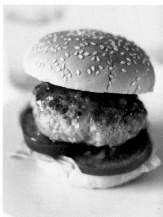

2.5cm/1in piece fresh root ginger, peeled
1 lemon grass stalk
2 spring onions (scallions)
450g/1lb minced (ground) pork
ground black pepper
30ml/2 tbsp sunflower oil
4 seeded bread rolls
2 tomatoes, sliced
8 cucumber slices
½ lettuce, shredded

1 Grate the ginger using a fine grater. Remove the tough outer layers from the lemon grass stalk and discard, then chop the centre finely. Finely chop the spring onions.

2 Combine the minced pork, pepper, ginger, lemon grass and onion. Shape into four patties with dampened hands, put on a plate and chill for 20 minutes.

3 Heat the oil in a non-stick griddle pan and cook the patties for 3–4 minutes on each side, until golden and cooked through.

4 Cut the bread rolls in half. Drain the patties on kitchen paper, then serve in the buns with the tomatoes, cucumber and lettuce.

Per portion Energy 477kcal/2007kJ; Protein 30.3g; Carbohydrate 44.5g, of which sugars 4.9g; Fat 21.1g, of which saturates 5.8g; Cholesterol 74mg; Calcium 133mg; Fibre 3.3g; Sodium 550mg.

477 calories

Cottage pie

You can't go wrong with a cottage pie – especially in the cold winter months, and this version is packed with hidden vegetables so it is a well-balanced meal in a bowl. Double the quantities if you want to freeze some portions for another time. You could use lean lamb instead of beef if you like, to make shepherd's pie.

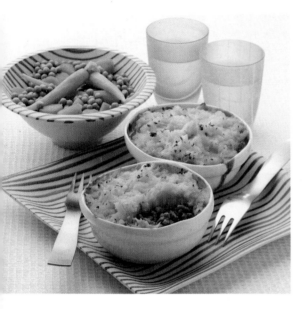

serves 4

1 small onion, peeled
350g/12oz lean minced (ground) beef
20ml/4 tsp plain (all-purpose) flour
30ml/2 tbsp reduced-salt and reduced-sugar
  tomato ketchup
300ml/½ pint/1¼ cups low-salt beef stock
a pinch of dried mixed herbs
salt and ground black pepper, to taste
115g/4oz swede (rutabaga), peeled
115g/4oz parsnip, peeled
2 potatoes, peeled
30ml/2 tbsp semi-skimmed (low-fat) milk
30ml/2 tbsp unsalted butter
cooked carrots and peas, to serve

1 Preheat the oven to 190°C/375°F/Gas 5. Finely chop the onion and place it in a large frying pan with the minced beef.

2 Over a low heat, dry-fry the meat and onion, stirring often, until it is evenly browned. The fat will render from the meat as it heats up, meaning no extra oil is required.

3 Add the flour, stirring, then add the ketchup, stock and herbs. Season to taste. Bring to the boil, reduce the heat, cover and simmer for 30 minutes, stirring often.

4 Chop the swede, parsnip and potato. Place the vegetables in a pan, cover with water and bring to the boil. Reduce the heat. Simmer for about 20 minutes, until tender.

5 Drain the vegetables in a colander. Return to the pan and mash them with the milk and half of the butter.

6 Spoon the meat into four small ovenproof dishes or one large one. Place the mashed root vegetables on top and fluff up with a fork. Dot with the remaining butter.

7 Place the dish or dishes on a baking sheet and cook for 25–30 minutes, until browned on top. Serve with cooked carrots and peas.

Per portion Energy 309kcal/1292kJ; Protein 21.9g; Carbohydrate 21.4g, of which sugars 7.2g; Fat 15.7g, of which saturates 7.9g; Cholesterol 82mg; Calcium 60mg; Fibre 3.7g; Sodium 264mg.

309
calories

Braised beef with vegetables

This one-pot dish is slowly cooked until the meat is meltingly tender, which is important if you want children to eat it since many do not like the texture of red meat. If they still turn up their noses at this, you can omit the potatoes, finely chop the vegetables and shred the meat with two forks to form a ragù that can be mixed with pasta.

serves 8

45ml/3 tbsp plain (all-purpose) flour
salt and ground black pepper, to taste
900g/2lb lean stewing steak, cut into
   5cm/2in cubes
45ml/3 tbsp oil
1 large onion, peeled and thinly sliced
1 large carrot, peeled and thickly sliced
2 celery sticks, finely chopped
300ml/½ pint/¼ cup low-salt beef stock
30ml/2 tbsp tomato purée (paste)
5ml/1 tsp dried mixed herbs
225g/8oz baby potatoes, halved
2 leeks, sliced

1 Preheat the oven to 150°C/300°F/Gas 2. Put the flour in a large bowl, season it, then add the beef cubes and toss to coat.

2 Heat the oil in a large, flameproof casserole. Add a small batch of meat, cook it quickly until it is browned on all sides and, with a slotted spoon, lift out. Repeat with the remaining beef.

3 Add the onion, carrot and celery to the casserole. Cook over medium heat for about 10 minutes, stirring frequently, until they begin to soften and brown slightly on the edges.

4 Return the meat to the casserole and add the stock, tomato purée and herbs, at the same time scraping up any sediment that has stuck to the bottom of the casserole. Heat until the liquid nearly comes to the boil.

5 Cover the casserole with a tight-fitting lid and put it into the hot oven. Cook for 2–2½ hours, or until the beef is tender.

6 Gently stir in the potatoes and leeks, cover and continue cooking for a further 30 minutes or until the potatoes are soft.

variation

• You could replace the beef with some lean stewing lamb, such as neck, if you like.

Per portion Energy 257kcal/1075kJ; Protein 27.9g; Carbohydrate 15.3g, of which sugars 5.2g; Fat 9.7g, of which saturates 2.7g; Cholesterol 75mg; Calcium 53mg; Fibre 3.3g; Sodium 95mg.

257 calories

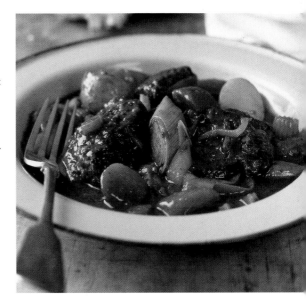

Spaghetti bolognese

A little smoked bacon seasons this classic meat sauce, meaning no additional salt is required. Porcini mushrooms add depth of flavour, while the passata and tomato paste intensify both the colour of the dish and its tomato taste. This dish is ideally suited to batch cooking, so make twice the amount and freeze half.

serves 4–6

25g/1oz dried porcini mushrooms (optional)
90ml/6 tbsp olive oil or vegetable oil
1 onion, peeled and finely chopped
2 celery sticks, finely chopped
1 carrot, peeled and finely chopped
1 garlic clove, peeled and finely chopped
50g/2oz smoked lean bacon, finely chopped
450g/1lb/2 cups lean minced (ground) beef
200ml/7fl oz/scant 1 cup low-salt beef stock
15ml/1 tsp tomato purée (paste) diluted with
   90ml/6 tbsp warm water
400g/14oz passata (bottled strained tomatoes)
   or canned chopped tomatoes
ground black pepper, to taste
400g/14oz spaghetti

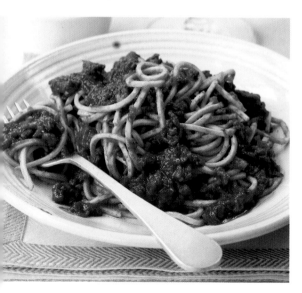

1 If using the porcini mushrooms, put them in a small bowl with warm water to cover and leave them to soak for 15 minutes, then drain. Discard the stems and slice the caps.

2 Heat the oil in a large, heavy pan and fry the onion, celery, carrot and garlic for 10 minutes, until the onion is soft and transparent.

3 Add the smoked lean bacon, stir to combine, and cook over low heat for 4 minutes more.

4 Add the porcini (if using) and the beef. Increase the heat to medium and brown the beef, without letting it go crisp, then pour in the beef stock.

5 Pour in the diluted tomato purée and the passata or canned tomatoes. Stir, season to taste, lower the heat and cover. Simmer very slowly for about 2 hours, stirring frequently and adding water or stock if the mixture becomes too thick.

6 Cook the spaghetti in a large pan of boiling water for 8–10 minutes, until al dente, then stir in the bolognese sauce and serve.

variation

• For a leaner bolognese, substitute minced (ground) pork, chicken or turkey for half of the minced beef.

Per portion Energy 509kcal/2141kJ; Protein 27.7g; Carbohydrate 55g, of which sugars 6.9g; Fat 21.4g, of which saturates 5.6g; Cholesterol 49mg; Calcium 47mg; Fibre 4.4g; Sodium 295mg.

509 calories

Pittas with lamb koftas

These slightly spicy koftas can be made in advance and stored in an airtight container for three days, ready for you to grill, broil or barbecue at a moment's notice.

serves 8

450g/1lb/2 cups minced (ground) lamb
salt and ground black pepper, to taste
1 small onion, peeled and finely chopped
10ml/2 tsp harissa paste (optional)
a small of handful fresh mint
150ml/¼ pint/⅔ cup low-fat natural (plain) yogurt
8 wholemeal (whole-wheat) pitta breads
cucumber and tomato slices, to serve

1 Prepare a barbecue or preheat the grill or broiler. Soak eight wooden skewers in cold water for about 1 hour to prevent them burning.

2 Meanwhile, mix together the lamb, seasoning, onion and harissa paste, if using. Divide the mixture into eight pieces and, using wet hands, press the meat on to the skewers in a sausage shape.

3 Heat for 10 minutes over the hot coals or under the grill, turning occasionally, until cooked.

4 Chop the mint and mix it with the yogurt. Season to taste and set aside. Warm the pitta breads on the barbecue or under the grill for a few seconds, then split in half.

5 Place a kofta in each pitta and remove the skewer. Add some cucumber and tomato slices. Drizzle with the yogurt sauce.

Per portion Energy 369kcal/1557kJ; Protein 20.6g; Carbohydrate 54.8g, of which sugars 4.8g; Fat 9g, of which saturates 3.8g; Cholesterol 44mg; Calcium 184mg; Fibre 2.4g; Sodium 469mg.

369
calories

Bulgur wheat with lamb

This is a complete meal in a bowl, and the secret to its low-fat status lies in the fact that only a small amount of meat is used, the bulk being supplied by bulgur.

serves 6

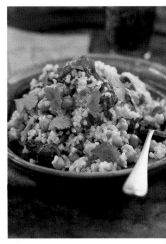

15ml/1 tbsp olive oil
1 onion, finely chopped
5ml/1 tsp ground cumin
200g/7oz lean lamb,
    cut into chunks
250g/9oz/1½ cups coarse
    bulgur wheat, rinsed
salt and ground black
    pepper, to taste
200g/7oz/1⅓ cups
    cooked chickpeas
fresh coriander (cilantro),
    to garnish

1 Heat the oil in a pan and add the onion. Cook, stirring, for 10 minutes. Stir in the ground cumin.

2 Toss the lamb into the pan and stir to coat in the onion and cumin. Add the bulgur wheat and about 900ml/1½ pints/3¾ cups water and bring to the boil. Season, then simmer for 20 minutes.

3 When all the water has been absorbed, turn off the heat, cover the pan with a dish towel and a lid, and leave to stand, undisturbed, for 10 minutes.

4 Fork through the mixture to separate the grains, then stir in the chickpeas. Serve, garnished with fresh coriander.

Per portion Energy 260kcal/1089kJ; Protein 13.5g; Carbohydrate 38.7g, of which sugars 1.3g; Fat 6.3g, of which saturates 1.5g; Cholesterol 25mg; Calcium 48mg; Fibre 2.2g; Sodium 100mg.

260
calories

DESSERTS

Coconut berry popsicles

These popsicles are perfect for children's parties and can be made in minutes! If you don't have much time, just use fresh berries without macerating them.

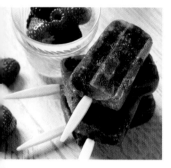

makes 10

350g/12oz/3 cups mixed fresh berries
60ml/4 tbsp clear honey (optional – omit if the berries are sweet)
250ml/8fl oz/1 cup coconut water

1 Hull the berries. If using strawberries, slice them into 5mm/¼in thick slices. Place in a dish and drizzle with the honey, if using. Pour over the coconut water. Leave to macerate in the refrigerator for at least 30 minutes, or up to 24 hours.

2 When you're ready to make the popsicles, remove the berries from the liquid with a fork. Drop the berries one by one into a 10–popsicle mould, layering them so the flat sides of the strawberries are pressed up against the edges of the mould. Arrange any whole berries to show them off as much as possible in the sides of the mould.

3 When all of the berries are in the moulds, carefully pour the liquid in to fill them.

4 Insert the sticks and freeze the popsicles for at least 1 hour. They will keep in the moulds for up to 6 months.

Per portion Energy 10kcal/41kJ; Protein 0.9g; Carbohydrate 1.4g, of which sugars 2.9g; Fat 0.1g, of which saturates 0g; Cholesterol 0mg; Calcium 8mg; Fibre 1.8g; Sodium 64mg.

10 calories

Summer berry frozen yogurt

Any combination of summer fruits will work for this deliciously creamy yet tangy dish, as long as they are frozen, because this helps to create a chunky texture.

serves 6

350g/12oz/3 cups frozen summer fruits, plus whole fresh or frozen berries, to decorate
200g/7oz/scant 1 cup low-fat natural (plain) yogurt
25g/1oz icing (confectioners') sugar

1 Put all the ingredients into a food processor and process until combined but still quite chunky. Spoon the mixture into six 150ml/¼ pint/⅔ cup ramekin dishes.

2 Cover each dish with clear film or plastic wrap and place in the freezer for about 2 hours, or until firm.

3 To turn out the frozen yogurts, dip the ramekin dishes briefly in hot water, taking care not to allow water to get on to the dessert itself. Invert the ramekins on to small serving plates. Tap the base of the dishes and the yogurts should come out fairly easily.

4 Serve immediately with fresh or frozen berries, such as blueberries, blackberries or raspberries.

variation

• To make a more creamy iced dessert, use Greek (US strained plain) yogurt. This will still be healthy, although slightly higher in fat.

Per portion Energy 51Kcal/215kJ; Protein 2.2g; Carbohydrate 10.4g, of which sugars 10.4g; Fat 0.4g, of which saturates 0.2g; Cholesterol 0mg; Calcium 75mg; Fibre 0.7g; Sodium 32mg.

51 calories

Instant ice creams

Nothing beats an ice cream on a hot day, but some are laden with sugar and fat. These healthy versions are a cinch to make and taste divine.

serves 4

banana ice cream
4 ripe bananas, peeled and sliced into chunks
60ml/4 tbsp semi-skimmed (low-fat) milk or low-fat natural (plain) yogurt

mixed berry ice cream
225g/8oz/2 cups frozen mixed berries
225g/8oz/1 cup low-fat natural (plain) yogurt
25g/1oz icing (confectioners') sugar

1 For the **banana ice cream**, place the bananas in a freezerproof container and freeze for 1 hour.

2 Transfer the frozen bananas to a blender or food processor with the milk or yogurt and blend until smooth. Serve immediately.

3 For the **mixed berry ice cream**, put the berries, yogurt and sugar in a blender or food processor and blend until smooth. Serve immediately.

cook's tip

• Rather than throwing out overripe bananas, peel and chop them and store them in the freezer.

Banana: **per portion** Energy 104kcal/439kJ; Protein 1.9g; Carbohydrate 24.3g, of which sugars 22g; Fat 0.5g, of which saturates 0.2g; Cholesterol 0mg; Calcium 30mg; Fibre 1.5g; Sodium 11mg.

104 calories

Mixed berry: **per portion** Energy 71kcal/303kJ; Protein 3.2g; Carbohydrate 14.2g, of which sugars 14.1g; Fat 0.6g, of which saturates 0.4g; Cholesterol 1mg; Calcium 100mg; Fibre 0.8g; Sodium 40mg.

71 calories

Grape jellies

Unlike chemical- and sugar-laden store-bought jellies, these rely on grape juice for colour and flavour. They need to be made a day in advance, in order to set.

serves 6

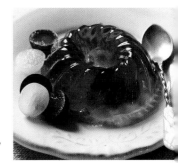

4 sheets unflavoured gelatine leaves, cut into quarters
400ml/14fl oz/1⅔ cups red grape juice
a bunch of red grapes, halved and deseeded, to serve

1 Soak the gelatine in the juice for 5–10 minutes in a heatproof bowl. Gently squeeze out the liquid from the gelatine then return to the bowl.

2 Position the heatproof bowl over a pan of barely simmering water. Do not let the bottom of the bowl touch the water. Slowly heat the juice over a low heat until very warm, but not boiling. Remove from the heat after about 10 minutes, when all of the gelatine has dissolved.

3 Pour the mixture into six individual silicone moulds standing on a plate, pouring slowly to avoid creating air bubbles. Carefully transfer to the refrigerator to set for at least 8 hours.

4 To remove the jellies from the moulds, suspend the bottom and sides of each of the moulds in warm water for 2–3 seconds. Invert on to serving plates, arrange the grapes on the plates and serve.

Per portion Energy 55kcal/233kJ; Protein 3.8g; Carbohydrate 10.4g, of which sugars 10.4g; Fat 0.1g, of which saturates 0g; Cholesterol 0mg; Calcium 25mg; Fibre 0.2g; Sodium 19mg.

55 calories

Fabulous fruit salad

Tropical fruit is perfect for picnic and packed-lunch fruit salads as it stays firm and fresh for quite a long time and always has a tasty, refreshing flavour.

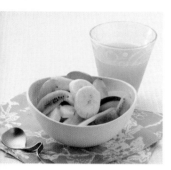

serves 4

1 small pineapple
2 kiwi fruit
1 ripe mango
1 slice watermelon
2 peaches
2 bananas
60ml/4 tbsp tropical
    fruit juice

1 Slice the base and top off the pineapple. Stand it upright. Cut away the skin and cut out the 'eyes' (dark round pieces). Cut the pineapple in half lengthways, then cut out the core. Chop the flesh into bitesize pieces and put them in a bowl.

2 Peel the skin from the kiwi. Cut it in half lengthways, then into wedges. Add to the bowl.

3 Peel the mango with a peeler, then stand it on a board and cut down to create slices. Cut these into smaller pieces. Cut the skin off the watermelon slice and discard it. Cut the flesh into chunks, then deseed.

4 Cut the peaches in half, remove the stones (pits) and cut into wedges. Peel then slice the bananas. Add all the fruit to the bowl and stir in the fruit juice. Cover with clear film or plastic wrap and chill for 30 minutes before serving.

Per portion Energy 162kcal/692kJ; Protein 2.4g; Carbohydrate 38.8g, of which sugars 37.5g; Fat 0.8g, of which saturates 0.2g; Cholesterol 0mg; Calcium 42mg; Fibre 4.1g; Sodium 8mg.

162 calories

Strawberry delight

The fragrant sauce brings out the sweetness of the strawberries in this delicious dessert, which tastes wonderful on its own or with some low-fat yogurt.

serves 4

350g/12oz/3 cups raspberries, fresh or frozen
15ml/1 tbsp clear honey
1 passion fruit
700g/1½lb/6 cups small strawberries

1 Place the raspberries and honey in a small pan and warm over a very gentle heat to release the juices. When the juices start to run, simmer for 5 minutes, stirring occasionally. Set aside and allow the mixture to cool.

2 Halve the passion fruit and, using a teaspoon, scoop the seeds and juice into a small bowl.

3 Put the raspberries into a food processor or blender, add the passion fruit and blend.

4 Place the raspberry and passion fruit sauce in a fine nylon sieve or strainer and press the purée through to remove the gritty seeds.

5 Divide the strawberries among serving bowls, spoon over some of the sauce and serve. Offer extra sauce separately, in a small jug or pitcher.

variation

• Try serving the sauce with a combination of soft fruits, such as peaches and bananas.

Per portion Energy 81kcal/345kJ; Protein 2.7g; Carbohydrate 17.6g, of which sugars 17.6g; Fat 0.5g, of which saturates 0.1g; Cholesterol 0mg; Calcium 51mg; Fibre 5.7g; Sodium 14mg.

81 calories

Apricot dessert

This quick and easy dessert uses dried, ready-to-eat apricots and coconut water, but mixed dried fruit such as apples, pears and peaches would also be good.

serves 6
. . . .

500g/1¼lb/2½ cups dried ready-to-eat apricots
600ml/1 pint/2½ cups coconut water
4 cloves
2 star anise
30ml/1 tbsp soft light brown sugar
30–45ml/2–3 tbsp lightly crushed toasted
   pistachio nuts, to garnish

1 Put the apricots into a pan with the coconut water and 150ml/¼ pint/⅔ cup water, the cloves and the star anise, and bring to the boil. Reduce the heat to low, cover the pan and simmer for 15 minutes, or until the apricots are soft and tender. Stir at least twice during this time to ensure even cooking.

2 Remove the spices from the pan and discard them. Remove half of the apricots with a slotted spoon and set aside. Purée the remainder, along with the cooking juices, and return the purée to the pan. Add the whole apricots.

3 Add the sugar and stir to combine. Cook gently for 3–4 minutes, then remove the pan from the heat and allow to cool for 30 minutes.

4 Divide the apricot mixture between four serving dishes, top with some crushed pistachio nuts and serve.

Per portion Energy 151kcal/646kJ; Protein 3.4g; Carbohydrate 35.6g, of which sugars 35.6g; Fat 0.5g, of which saturates 0g; Cholesterol 0mg; Calcium 62mg; Fibre 7g; Sodium 12mg.

151 calories

Fruit fondue

This dessert is great for enticing children to eat lots of fruit. Make sure the melted chocolate has cooled to room temperature before mixing it into the yogurt.

serves 6
. . . .

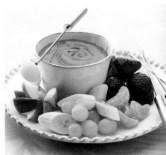

40g/1½oz milk chocolate
a selection of fruit, such as
   apples, bananas,
   satsumas, strawberries
   and grapes
200g/7oz/1 cup full-fat
   Greek (US whole
   strained plain) yogurt

1 Break up the chocolate and place it in a heatproof bowl set over a pan of just simmering water, until melted. Leave to cool to room temperature, or lumps of chocolate will form when you stir it into the yogurt.

2 Meanwhile, cut the apple into quarters. Cut away the core and then cut the apple into bitesize pieces. Slice the bananas thickly and break the satsumas into segments. Remove the stalks and leaves from the strawberries by twisting and pulling them out. Break the grapes off their stalks.

3 Whisk the yogurt in a serving bowl, then quickly stir in the melted chocolate. It doesn't matter too much if a few lumps of chocolate do form.

4 Stand the bowl on a large plate and arrange the fruit around the bowl. Serve with fondue forks or standard forks for spearing and dipping the fruit.

Per portion Energy 172kcal/726kJ; Protein 3.7g; Carbohydrate 28.3g, of which sugars 27.3g; Fat 5.7g, of which saturates 3.5g; Cholesterol 7mg; Calcium 77mg; Fibre 3g; Sodium 33mg.

172 calories

Superberry semolina

Berries are a fabulous addition to traditional desserts such as semolina. This whisked version is light and, with the amazing colour of the berries, will look stunning too.

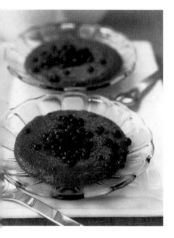

serves 4

1 litre/1¾ pints/4 cups water
300g/11oz bilberries, cranberries, blackcurrants or raspberries
150g/5oz/scant 1 cup semolina
45ml/3 tbsp clear honey, or to taste
fresh berries, to decorate

1 Put the water and berries in a pan and bring to the boil. Strain the liquid into a clean pan. Discard the berries or strain them into the liquid.

2 Put the semolina in the pan and, stirring all the time, return to the boil. Reduce the heat and simmer for 5 minutes, until the semolina is cooked. Add the honey according to taste and the type of fruit used.

3 Turn the mixture into a bowl and whisk for at least 5 minutes using an electric whisk, until light and frothy.

4 Divide the mixture among individual serving bowls and sprinkle over a few berries to decorate.

Per portion Energy 183kcal/779kJ; Protein 5.1g; Carbohydrate 41.1g, of which sugars 12.1g; Fat 0.9g, of which saturates 0.1g; Cholesterol 0mg; Calcium 26mg; Fibre 3.6g; Sodium 8mg.

183 calories

Rice pudding

This dessert is nutritious, warming and so easy to make. You can add dried fruits and chopped nuts to the mixture if you like, and serve it with fruit compote.

serves 6

non-stick baking oil, for greasing
50g/2oz/¼ cup pudding rice
30ml/2 tbsp soft light brown sugar
900ml/1½ pints/3¾ cups semi-skimmed (low-fat) milk or nut milk
small strip of lemon rind
freshly grated nutmeg

1 Preheat the oven to 150°C/300°F/Gas 2. Lightly grease a 1.2 litre/2 pint/5 cup shallow ovenproof dish with non-stick baking oil.

2 Put the rice and sugar into the dish and stir in the milk. Add the strip of lemon rind and sprinkle a little nutmeg over the surface. Put the pudding into the hot oven.

3 Cook the pudding for about 2 hours, stirring after 30 minutes and another couple of times during the next 1½ hours, until the rice is tender and the pudding is thick and creamy.

4 If you prefer skin on top, leave the pudding undisturbed for the final 30 minutes; or stir again.

cook's tip

• Nut milk, especially hazelnut milk, lends a lovely flavour to the dessert, along with nutrients.

Per portion Energy 119kcal/500kJ; Protein 5.6g; Carbohydrate 19.2g, of which sugars 12.6g; Fat 2.5g, of which saturates 1.7g; Cholesterol 11mg; Calcium 168mg; Fibre 0g; Sodium 75mg.

119 calories

Baked apple pudding

This soft, soufflé-like dessert is naturally sweetened by apples and is packed with nutrition. Soft or stewed fruit would also make a good base for this dessert.

serves 4

4 crisp eating apples, peeled, cored and sliced
    and sprinkled with a little lemon juice
300ml/½ pint/1¼ cups semi-skimmed (low-fat) milk
40g/1½oz/3 tbsp unsalted butter, plus extra
    for greasing
40g/1½oz/⅓ cup plain (all-purpose) flour
15ml/1 tbsp caster (superfine) sugar
2.5ml/½ tsp vanilla extract
2 eggs, separated

1 Preheat the oven to 200°C/400°F/Gas 6. Butter a dish measuring 20–23cm/8–9in diameter and 5cm/2in deep. Arrange the apples in the dish.

2 Put the milk, butter and flour in a pan. Stirring continuously with a whisk, cook over medium heat until the sauce thickens and comes to the boil. Let it bubble gently for 1–2 minutes, stirring well to make sure it does not stick and burn on the bottom of the pan. Pour into a bowl, add the sugar and vanilla, and then stir in the egg yolks.

3 In a separate bowl, whisk the egg whites until stiff peaks form. With a large metal spoon, fold the egg whites into the custard. Pour over the apples.

4 Put the dish into the hot oven and cook for about 40 minutes, until puffed up, deep golden brown and firm to the touch. Serve immediately.

Per portion Energy 250kcal/1047kJ; Protein 7.7g; Carbohydrate 27.2g, of which sugars 19.6g; Fat 13g, of which saturates 7g; Cholesterol 142mg; Calcium 121mg; Fibre 2.8g; Sodium 144mg.

250 calories

Hedgerow crumble

Crumbles are a wonderful way to present fruit to children, and this topping is made with wholemeal flour and oatmeal for added goodness.

serves 8

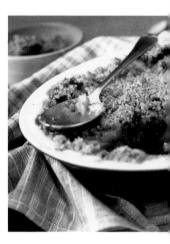

115g/4oz/½ cup
    unsalted butter
115g/4oz/1 cup
    wholemeal (whole-
    wheat) flour
50g/2oz/½ cup oatmeal
75g/3oz/6 tbsp cup soft
    light brown sugar
900g/2lb cooking apples
450g/1lb/4 cups
    blackberries
    (or raspberries)

1 Preheat the oven to 190°C/375°F/Gas 5. To make the crumble, rub the butter into the flour, until it resembles fine breadcrumbs.

2 Add the oatmeal and 30ml/2 tbsp brown sugar and continue to rub in until the mixture begins to stick together, forming large crumbs.

3 Peel, core and slice the cooking apples and place the apples, berries, 30ml/2 tbsp water and remaining sugar in a shallow ovenproof dish, about 2 litres/3½ pints/9 cups capacity.

4 Cover the fruit with the crumble topping. Put into the hot oven and cook for 30–40 minutes, until the fruit is soft and the top is golden brown.

Per portion Energy 267kcal/1121kJ; Protein 3.6g; Carbohydrate 36.5g, of which sugars 23.1g; Fat 12.9g, of which saturates 7.5g; Cholesterol 31mg; Calcium 42mg; Fibre 7g; Sodium 94mg.

267 calories

SWEET TREATS

Fruity flapjacks

These flapjacks are free of refined sugar, and lower in fat than standard ones. Sugar comes in the form of fructose, and less is needed than if you were to use refined.

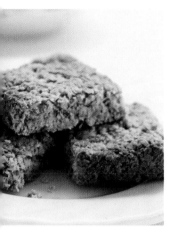

makes 9

75g/3oz/¾ cup ready-
  to-eat dried apricots,
  finely chopped
1 eating apple, cored
  and grated
150g/5oz/1¼ cups
  unsweetened Swiss-
  style muesli (granola)
150ml/¼ pint/⅔ cup
  apple juice
15g/½oz/1 tbsp soft
  sunflower margarine

1 Preheat the oven to 190°C/375°F/Gas 5. Use a tiny amount of spray oil to grease an 18 x 18cm/7 x 7in square tin or pan.

2 Mix together all of the ingredients in a large bowl with a wooden spoon.

3 Press the mixture into the prepared tin or pan and bake for 35–40 minutes, or until the surface is lightly browned and firm.

4 Mark into nine squares with the blade of a knife and leave to cool completely in the tin or pan.

5 Turn out the flapjack and cut or break along the scored lines. Store in an airtight container.

Per portion Energy 110Kcal/465kJ; Protein 2g; Carbohydrate 20g, of which sugars 12g; Fat 3g, of which saturates 0g; Cholesterol 0mg; Calcium 29mg; Fibre 3g; Sodium 86mg.

110
calories

Date and muesli slice

Made up of oats, seeds, dates, raisins and natural yogurt, these low-fat bars are a supernutrient-packed treat to add to a lunchbox or picnic.

serves 12–16

175g/6oz/¾ cup light muscovado (brown) sugar
175g/6oz/1 cup ready-to-eat dried dates, chopped
115g/4oz/1 cup self-raising (self-rising) flour
50g/2oz/½ cup muesli (granola)
30ml/2 tbsp sunflower seeds
15ml/1 tbsp poppy seeds
30ml/2 tbsp sultanas (golden raisins)
150ml/¼ pint/⅔ cup low-fat natural (plain) yogurt
1 egg, beaten

1 Preheat the oven to 180°C/350°F/Gas 4. Line a 28 x 18cm/11 x 7in shallow baking tin or pan with baking parchment.

2 Mix together all the ingredients in a large bowl until thoroughly combined.

3 Spread the mixture evenly in the tin or pan and bake for 25 minutes, until golden brown.

4 Remove from the oven and allow to cool before cutting into squares and serving.

variation
• Coconut palm sugar has a very similar flavour and consistency to light muscovado (brown) sugar, but it is low-GI and packed with vitamins and minerals. It makes a great healthier substitute and is available in health-food stores or online.

Per portion Energy 135kcal/572kJ; Protein 2.9g; Carbohydrate 28.8g, of which sugars 21.5g; Fat 2.2g, of which saturates 0.4g; Cholesterol 15mg; Calcium 70mg; Fibre 1.4g; Sodium 41mg.

135
calories

Almond and carrot bars

Carrot cake becomes a cookie bar in this more portable version, and is a great way to add to the fruit and vegetable count of children's lunchboxes. The wholemeal pastry base can be used as an alternative to standard pastry in many other sweet bakes, and you could omit the orange rind and create a savoury version, too.

makes 16

75g/3oz/6 tbsp unsalted butter, softened
150g/5oz/1¼ cups plain wholemeal (all-purpose whole-wheat) flour
finely grated rind of 1 orange

For the filling
90g/3½oz/7 tbsp unsalted butter, diced
75g/3oz/scant ½ cup caster (superfine) sugar
2 eggs
2.5ml/½ tsp almond extract
175g/6oz/1½ cups ground almonds
1 large cooked carrot, peeled and finely chopped

For the topping
175g/6oz/¾ cup low-fat cream cheese
30–45ml/2–3 tbsp chopped walnuts

1 Preheat the oven to 190°C/375°F/Gas 5. Lightly grease the base and sides of a 28 x 18cm/11 x 7in shallow baking tin or pan.

2 Put the butter, flour and orange rind into a bowl and rub together until the mixture resembles coarse breadcrumbs.

3 Add water, a teaspoon at a time, to mix to a firm but not sticky dough. Roll out on a floured surface and use to line the base of the tin or pan.

4 To make the filling, cream the butter and sugar together. Beat in the eggs and almond extract. Stir in the ground almonds and the finely chopped carrot to combine.

5 Spread the mixture over the dough base and bake for about 25 minutes or until it is firm in the centre and golden brown. Leave to cool completely in the tin or pan.

6 To make the topping, beat the cream cheese until smooth and spread it over the cooled, cooked filling. Swirl with a small palette knife or metal spatula, and sprinkle with the chopped walnuts. Cut into bars with a sharp knife.

Per portion Energy 231kcal/961kJ; Protein 6.4g; Carbohydrate 12.2g, of which sugars 6.1g; Fat 17.8g, of which saturates 6.8g; Cholesterol 53mg; Calcium 52mg; Fibre 1.2g; Sodium 123mg.

231 calories

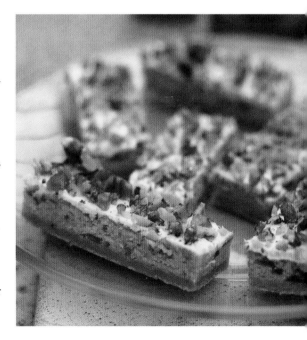

Orange oaties

These coconutty cookies are so delicious that it is difficult to believe that they are healthy too. Flavoursome and wonderfully crunchy, the whole family will love them.

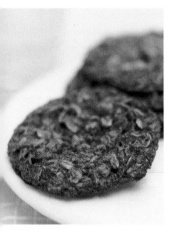

makes 16
• • • • • • • • • • • •

175g/6oz/¾ cup honey
120ml/4fl oz/½ cup
   coconut water
90g/3½oz/1 cup rolled
   oats, lightly toasted
115g/4oz/1 cup plain
   (all-purpose) flour
115g/4oz/½ cup caster
   (superfine) sugar
grated rind of 1 orange
5ml/1 tsp bicarbonate
   of soda (baking soda)

1 Preheat the oven to 180°C/350°F/Gas 4. Line two baking sheets with baking parchment.

2 Put the honey and coconut water in a small pan and simmer over a low heat for 8–10 minutes, stirring occasionally, until the mixture is thick.

3 Put the oats, flour, sugar and orange rind into a bowl. Mix the bicarbonate of soda with 15ml/ 1 tbsp boiling water and stir into the flour mixture, together with the honey syrup.

4 Place spoonfuls on to the baking sheets, spaced slightly apart, and bake for 10–12 minutes, until golden brown. Leave to cool on the sheets for 5 minutes, then transfer to a wire rack to cool.

Per portion Energy 104kcal/442kJ; Protein 1.6g; Carbohydrate 24.6g, of which sugars 15.4g; Fat 0.6g, of which saturates 0g; Cholesterol 0mg; Calcium 16mg; Fibre 1g; Sodium 108mg.

104
• • • • •
calories

Orange and apple rockies

You may know these classic cakes as 'rock' cakes. They are a fantastic low-fat teatime treat to throw together at a moment's notice. They are best served warm.

makes 24
• • • • • • • • • • • •

225g/8oz/2 cups self-raising (self-rising) flour
115g/4oz/½ cup hard baking margarine
oil, for greasing
1 large eating apple, peeled and quartered
50g/2oz/⅓ cup ready-to-eat dried apricots, chopped
50g/2oz/⅓ cup sultanas (golden raisins)
grated rind of 1 small orange
45ml/3 tbsp demerara (raw) sugar
1 egg
15ml/1 tbsp semi-skimmed (low-fat) milk

1 Put the flour into a large mixing bowl and rub in the margarine with your fingertips until the mixture resembles breadcrumbs. Set aside.

2 Preheat the oven to 190°C/375°F/Gas 5 and brush two baking sheets with a little oil.

3 Stir the apple and apricots into the flour mixture with the sultanas and orange rind. Stir the demerara sugar into the mixture.

4 Beat the egg and milk, then stir into the flour mixture until just beginning to bind together.

5 Drop spoonfuls, well spaced apart, on to the baking sheets. Bake for 12–15 minutes, until golden and firm. Transfer to a wire rack to cool slightly. Serve warm.

Per portion Energy 88kcal/368kJ; Protein 1.4g; Carbohydrate 11.4g, of which sugars 4.4g; Fat 4.4g, of which saturates 0.9g; Cholesterol 10mg; Calcium 39mg; Fibre 0.9g; Sodium 71mg.

88
• • • • •
calories

Banana muffins

Don't throw out nearly black bananas lurking in the fruit bowl – they will be perfect for these moist muffins, which contain just a little unrefined sugar. If you don't want to make the muffins immediately, you can peel the bananas, put them in a container and freeze them; then defrost and use them to make the recipe when you do have time.

makes 16

115g/4oz/1 cup plain (all-purpose) flour
115g/4oz/1 cup plain wholemeal (all-purpose whole-wheat) flour
5ml/1 tsp baking powder
5ml/1 tsp bicarbonate of soda (baking soda)
a pinch of salt
2.5ml/½ tsp ground cinnamon
1.5ml/¼ tsp ground nutmeg
3 large ripe bananas
1 egg
50g/2oz/¼ cup soft dark brown sugar
50ml/2fl oz/¼ cup vegetable oil
40g/1½oz/⅓ cup raisins

1 Preheat the oven to 190°C/375°F/Gas 5. Line a 16-hole cupcake tin or pan with paper cases.

2 Sift the flours, baking powder, bicarbonate of soda, salt, cinnamon and nutmeg into a large mixing bowl, lifting the sieve or strainer high. Set aside.

3 Put the bananas in a separate bowl and mash to a fine pulp with a fork or a wooden spoon.

4 Add the egg, sugar and oil to the bananas and beat with a wooden spoon to combine thoroughly.

5 Add the dry ingredients to the banana mixture and gently beat in gradually with a wooden spoon. Don't over-mix – the batter should look a bit 'knobbly'.

6 With the wooden spoon, gently stir in the raisins until just combined. Do not over-mix.

7 Spoon the mixture into the paper cases using metal spoons. Fill each one about two-thirds full. Bake for 15–20 minutes, until the tops spring back when touched with your finger. Remove from the oven, cool slightly in the tin or pan, then transfer to a wire rack to cool completely.

variation

• You could also add a spoonful of linseeds, fine oatmeal or rolled oats to the mixture.

Per portion Energy 112kcal/473kJ; Protein 2.4g; Carbohydrate 20.5g, of which sugars 10g; Fat 2.9g, of which saturates 0.5g; Cholesterol 14mg; Calcium 22mg; Fibre 1.6g; Sodium 106mg.

112 calories

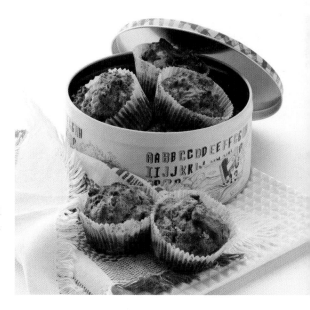

Peanut butter teabread

Crunchy peanut butter gives this teabread richness as well as a distinctive flavour and texture. It also adds protein, making this cake a substantial snack.

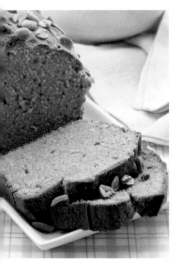

serves 10

225g/8oz/2 cups plain
  (all-purpose) flour
10ml/2 tsp baking
  powder
50g/2oz/¼ cup unsalted
  butter, softened
175g/6oz/½ cup
  sugar-free no-salt
  crunchy peanut butter
50g/2oz/¼ cup caster
  (superfine) sugar
2 eggs, beaten
250ml/8fl oz/1 cup
  semi-skimmed milk

1 Preheat the oven to 180°C/350°F/Gas 4. Line a 900g/2lb loaf tin or pan with baking parchment.

2 Sift the flour and baking powder together into a large bowl.

3 Beat the butter and peanut butter in a bowl to soften, then beat in the sugar until light and fluffy. Gradually whisk in the eggs a little at a time, then beat in the milk with the sifted flour.

4 Pour into the tin and bake for 1 hour, until a skewer comes out clean. Leave to cool in the tin for 5 minutes, then turn out on to a wire rack.

Per portion Energy 271kcal/1134kJ; Protein 8.5g; Carbohydrate 26.6g, of which sugars 8g; Fat 15.2g, of which saturates 5.5g; Cholesterol 59mg; Calcium 86mg; Fibre 0.9g; Sodium 240mg.

271 calories

Fruity carrot cake

This moist cake is packed with goodness, containing not only carrots but also bananas and figs, which add natural sweetness and flavour as well as fibre.

serves 10–12

225g/8oz/2 cups self-raising (self-rising) flour
10ml/2 tsp baking powder
150g/5oz/scant 1 cup soft light brown sugar
115g/4oz/⅔ cup ready-to-eat dried figs, chopped
225g/8oz carrots, peeled and grated
2 small ripe bananas, peeled and mashed
2 eggs
150ml/¼ pint/⅔ cup sunflower oil, plus extra
  for greasing

1 Grease and line an 18cm/7in cake tin or pan. Preheat the oven to 180°C/350°F/Gas 4.

2 Sift the flour, baking powder and sugar into a large bowl. Mix well, then stir in the figs.

3 Using your hands, squeeze as much liquid out of the grated carrots as you can, then add the carrot to the flour mixture. Add the bananas and stir to combine.

4 Lightly beat the eggs and oil together in a small mixing bowl with a fork, then pour them into the flour mixture. Beat well with a wooden spoon.

5 Transfer to the tin and level the top. Cook for 1–1¼ hours, until a skewer comes out clean. Leave to cool in the tin for 5 minutes, then turn out the cake on to a wire rack.

Per portion Energy 251kcal/1055kJ; Protein 3.6g; Carbohydrate 37.2g, of which sugars 22.6g; Fat 10.8g, of which saturates 1.5g; Cholesterol 39mg; Calcium 114mg; Fibre 2.5g; Sodium 191mg.

251 calories

Low-fat brownies

Brownies are always a hit, and keep well too. Unfortunately, most recipes are packed with fat, sugar and chocolate, which is not an ideal combination for anyone, let alone someone who is trying to manage their weight. These relatively healthy brownies taste just as good and contain fibre and vitamins to boot.

makes 9

75ml/5 tbsp reduced-fat cocoa powder
15ml/1 tbsp caster (superfine) sugar
75ml/5 tbsp skimmed milk
3 large bananas, mashed
175g/6oz/1 cup soft light brown sugar
5ml/1 tsp vanilla extract
5 egg whites
75g/3oz/¾ cup self-raising (self-rising) flour
75g/3oz/¾ cup oat bran
5ml/1 tsp icing (confectioners') sugar,
    for dusting (optional)

1 Preheat the oven to 180°C/350°F/Gas 4. Line a 20cm/8in square cake tin or pan with some baking parchment.

2 Blend the cocoa powder and caster sugar with the milk in a bowl. Mix in the bananas, soft light brown sugar and vanilla extract.

3 In a separate bowl, lightly beat the egg whites with a fork.

4 Add the chocolate mixture to the egg whites and continue to beat well. Sift the flour over the mixture and fold it in with the oat bran. Pour the mixture into the prepared tin.

5 Bake the brownie for 40 minutes or until the top is firm and crusty. Leave to cool in the tin before turning out and cutting into squares. Lightly dust the brownies with a little icing sugar if you like, before serving.

cook's tips

• Make sure the bananas are ripe, as under-ripe ones will be less sweet and harder to mash.
• It is important not to over-cook brownies, or they will be dry. The top should be just firm, but the mixture underneath should have a bit of a wobble. They will set as they cool.
• Don't be tempted to swap wholemeal (wholewheat) flour for the white flour used here, or the brownies will be too dense and chewy.

Per portion Energy 101kcal/426kJ; Protein 4.6g; Carbohydrate 16.6g, of which sugars 10.8g; Fat 2.2g, of which saturates 1.2g; Cholesterol 0mg; Calcium 31mg; Fibre 2.8g; Sodium 167mg.

101 calories

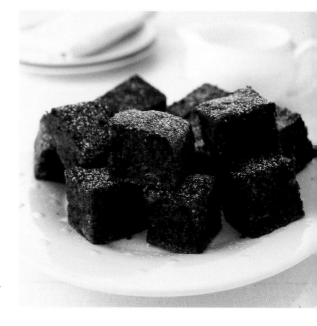

Snowmen pops

These tiny pops, made from fat-free meringues with a chewy centre, are quick and easy to prepare and look wonderful. While they are not exactly nutritious, meringues are much lower in calories than many other festive foods and every child deserves the odd treat.

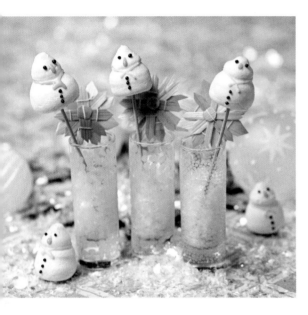

makes 25

2 egg whites
115g/4oz/generous ½ cup caster (superfine) sugar
100g/3¾oz/scant 1 cup fondant icing
   (confectioners') sugar
15–30ml/1–2 tbsp water
a few drops of black, orange and blue food
   colouring gels

1 Preheat the oven to 140°C/275°F/Gas 1. Line two baking sheets with baking parchment.

2 Whisk the egg whites until they hold stiff peaks. Gradually add the caster sugar, a tablespoonful at a time, whisking constantly until the meringue is thick, shiny and glossy.

3 Using a piping (pastry) bag fitted with a large plain nozzle, pipe 25 3cm/1¼in-diameter rounds on to the baking sheets. Pipe a second, smaller round on top of each one to give a snowman shape, with a round body and smaller head.

4 Smooth the top of the second round using a clean finger. Bake for 1–1¼ hours, or until the meringues are dried and crisp. Leave them to cool completely on the baking sheets.

5 Sift the fondant icing sugar into a bowl and stir in enough water to give a smooth, thick icing. Divide the icing among three bowls and add black food colouring gel to one, orange to another and blue to the third.

6 Using three separate piping bags, each fitted with a very small plain nozzle, pipe a small orange carrot nose, a thin blue scarf, three black buttons and two black eyes on to each snowman.

7 Leave the icing to set, then insert a wooden skewer into the base of each snowman. Stand the pops in a tall glass, or you can insert them into some florist's foam covered in silver paper.

cook's tip

• Meringues store extremely well in an airtight container, so these are brilliant make-ahead bakes. Just add the skewers at the last minute.

Per portion Nutritional information: Energy 35kcal/ 148kJ; Protein 0g; Carbohydrate 9g, of which sugars 9g; Fat 0g, of which saturates 0g; Cholesterol 0mg; Calcium 1mg; Fibre 0g; Sodium 6mg.

35 calories

Marshmallow daisy cakes

These are quick and simple to make and contain relatively few calories compared with most treats; you can also leave off the marshmallows if you prefer. By making individual cakes, you can control portions accurately, and it is likely that there will be less waste.

makes 12

115g/4oz/1 cup self-raising (self-rising) flour
5ml/1 tsp baking powder
115g/4oz/generous ½ cup caster (superfine) sugar
115g/4oz/½ cup soft baking margarine
2 large (US extra large) eggs, beaten
15ml/1 tbsp lemon juice
finely grated rind of 1 lemon

For the decoration
50g/2oz/¼ cup unsalted butter
115g/4oz/1 cup icing (confectioners') sugar, sifted
5ml/1 tsp lemon juice
12 pink and white marshmallows
12 small sweets or candies

1 Preheat the oven to 180°C/350°F/Gas 4. Line a 12-cup muffin tin or pan with paper cases.

2 Sift the flour and baking powder into a large bowl, then add the remaining ingredients. Beat until light and creamy, then place heaped spoonfuls into the paper cases.

3 Bake for about 20 minutes, or until golden and firm to the touch. Allow to cool for 2 minutes, then turn out on to a wire rack to go cold.

4 For the decoration, beat the butter with a wooden spoon until it is soft and pale, then add the sifted icing sugar and 5ml/1 tsp lemon juice to make a smooth buttercream.

5 Spread the top of each completely cooled cake with a little of the buttercream.

6 For the flower topping, use kitchen scissors to cut each marshmallow in half horizontally. Then cut in half again to create semicircles. Press the tips of each set of four semicircles together to form four petals of a flower. Arrange these on top of each cupcake and press a sweet into the centre.

variation

• These light little cakes are still delicious without the icing and decorations, for a lower-sugar snack.

Per portion Energy 235kcal/983kJ; Protein 2.5g; Carbohydrate 29.2g, of which sugars 21.5g; Fat 12.8g, of which saturates 4.2g; Cholesterol 54mg; Calcium 48mg; Fibre 0.4g; Sodium 183mg.

235 calories

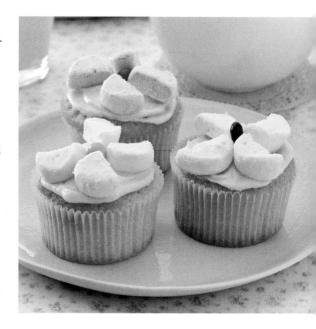

DIARIES AND PLANNERS

Food diary

NAME/DATE: . . . .

	REASON FOR EATING	WHAT WAS EATEN
MONDAY Time: Time: Time: Time:		
TUESDAY Time: Time: Time: Time:		
WEDNESDAY Time: Time: Time: Time:		
THURSDAY Time: Time: Time: Time:		
FRIDAY Time: Time: Time: Time:		
SATURDAY Time: Time: Time: Time:		
SUNDAY Time: Time: Time: Time:		

Menu planner

	BREAKFAST	SNACK OR DRINK	LUNCH	SNACK OR DRINK	DINNER
MONDAY					
TUESDAY					
WEDNESDAY					
THURSDAY					
FRIDAY					
SATURDAY					
SUNDAY					

Activity and screentime diary

	CHILD 1	CHILD 2	PARENT	PARENT
MONDAY Activity				
Screentime				
TUESDAY Activity				
Screentime				
WEDNESDAY Activity				
Screentime				
THURSDAY Activity				
Screentime				
FRIDAY Activity				
Screentime				
SATURDAY Activity				
Screentime				
SUNDAY Activity				
Screentime				

Family activity organizer

	WHAT	WHEN	WHO	TICK?
MONDAY				
TUESDAY				
WEDNESDAY				
THURSDAY				
FRIDAY				
SATURDAY				
SUNDAY				

INDEX

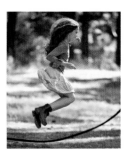

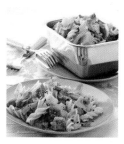

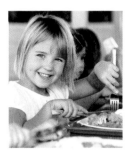